Raising Resilience

Take the stress out of feeding your family and love your life

36 WAYS TO HELP YOUR KIDS RELAX, LEARN, AND GROW

Including *Recipes for Resilience*

Jess Sherman, MEd, RHN

IC PUBLISHING

Copyright © 2016 Jessica Sherman

First published in Canada by I C Publishing 2016
Second printing, 2017
Third printing, 2019

All rights reserved. The use of any part of this publication reproduced, transmitted in any form or by any means, electronic, mechanical, photocopying, recording, or otherwise, or stored in a retrieval system, without the prior written consent of the author and publisher is an infringement of the copyright law. Your support of the author's rights is appreciated.

Library and Archives Canada Cataloguing in Publication

Sherman, Jessica, 1972-, author
Raising resilience : take the stress out of feeding your family &
love your life / Jessica Sherman.

Issued in print and electronic formats.
ISBN 978-1-927952-43-6 (paperback).—ISBN 978-1-927952-44-3 (pdf)

1. Children—Nutrition. 2. Nutrition. I. Title.

RJ206.S53 2016   613.2083   C2016-902480-6
C2016-902481-4

Although the author and publisher have made every effort to ensure that the information in this book was correct at press time, the author and publisher do not assume and hereby disclaim any liability to any party for any loss, damage or disruption caused by errors or omissions, whether such errors or omissions result from negligence, accident, or any other cause.

Publishing: I C Publishing
Production: WeMakeBooks.ca
Cover photo: Christin Gasner

Printed in Canada
ICpublishing.ca

Dear Reader

The purpose of this publication is to provide information and is not intended to be medical advice. The author is not a doctor and does not claim to be one. All suggestions and charts are meant as guides to give the reader insight into their child's health, but are not sufficient to diagnose medical conditions or create a treatment plan. Every child is unique and reacts differently to a range of foods. The use of supplements, though addressed in this book, should be discussed with a qualified practitioner, as individual needs may vary. The reader should consult with their health care teams before adopting suggestions in this book, and ultimately holds sole responsibility for the final decisions about how best to care for the health of their child/children.

TABLE OF CONTENTS

A MESSAGE TO THE READER 9
ACKNOWLEDGMENTS 13
INTRODUCTION 15
THE ROOTS OF RESILIENCE 15
    Healthy Resilience 17
    Success Stories 19
        Manny: 19
        Maggie: 20
HOW TO USE THIS BOOK 23
PART ONE: UNDERSTANDING DIMINISHED RESILIENCE 27
    Section Overview 27
    Removing Roadblocks 28
    Understanding Stress 30
    Identifying and Reducing Stressors in Children 35
        Social Stress 35
        Environmental Stress 37
        Biological Stress 38
    Top Biological Stressors 39
        Sugar 39
        Environmental Toxins 43
        Genetically Modified Foods (GMs or GMOs) 46
        Candida Yeast 46
        Adverse Food Reactions 48
        Additives 50
        Lack of Sleep 53
    Section Summary 55
PART TWO: THREE CORE DIETARY STRATEGIES FOR RAISING RESILIENCE 57
    Introduction to Core Dietary Strategies 57
    Core Strategy #1: Maximize Nutrient Density 58
        Section Overview 58
        The Power of Nutrients 58
        Nutrient Density 62
        Nutrient Categories 63
        Healthy Fat 65

Raising Resilience

  Fifteen Ways to Maximize Nutrient Density 75
 Section Summary 85
 Core Strategy #2: Control Blood Sugar 87
  Section Overview 87
  Understanding Carbohydrates 87
  Why is Blood Sugar Erratic and What Can You Do About It? 91
  Symptoms of Hypoglycemia (low blood sugar) 91
  Twelve Ways to Control Blood Sugar Fluctuations 93
 Section Summary 107
 Core Strategy #3: Support Digestion 108
  Section Overview 108
  Understanding the Digestive System 109
  Nine Ways to Support Your Child's Digestion 122
 Part Two Summary 134
  36 Ways to Help Your Child Relax, Learn, and Grow 134
PART THREE: SELF-REGULATION AND ENVIRONMENT 137
 Section Overview 137
 Positive Food Relationships 137
  Five Tips for Fostering a Positive Relationship with Food 139
  Managing Picky Eaters 144
  The Influence of Sensory Misreading and Poor Oral Motor Skills 154
 Section Summary 154
PART FOUR: TRANSITIONING TO RESILIENCE: FINDING YOUR 80/20 157
 The 80/20 Rule 157
 Your Plan For Transformation 161
CLOSING THOUGHTS 167
RECIPES FOR RESILIENCE 169
 A few words about these recipes 169
 A few notes about ingredients 169
 STAPLES 170
  Basic Ketchup 170
  Mayonnaise 171
  Chicken Broth 171
  Chicken Bone Stock 172
  Vegetable Stock 173
  Corn-Free Baking Powder 173
  Egg Replacers 174
  Fortified Salt 174
 BREAKFASTS 174
  Basic Breakfast Smoothie 174
  Pumpkin Power French Toast 175
  Rice/Millet Pudding 175
  Oven Oatmeal/Quinoa 176
  Quick and Easy Pumpkin Custard 177
  Protein-Packed Gluten-Free Pancakes 177

Table of Contents

SOUPS/SALADS 178
    Curried Squash-Lentil Soup 178
    Root Vegetable Soup 179
    Fortified Pesto-Arame Salad 179
    Cameron's Salad 180
WRAPS, DIPS & SPREADS 181
    Veggie Pâté 181
    Black Bean Wraps 181
    Hummus 3 Ways 182
    Citrus Guacamole 183
MAIN MEALS 184
    Lazy Cabbage Rolls 184
    Quick & Easy Fish Patties 184
    Quick Chicken Curry 185
    Mac and Cheese (dairy-free option) 185
SNACKS/TREATS 186
    Coconut-Chia Mango Pudding 186
    Gluten-Free Muffins 187
    Homemade Jello 188
    Grain-Free Banana Date Muffins 188
    Black Bean Brownies 189
    Golden Tea (Turmeric Tea) 190
    Digestive Tea 190
FABULOUS FERMENTS 191
    Basic Brine 191
    Fermented Carrot Sticks 191
    Fermented Ketchup 192
    Probiotic Lemonade 192
    Basic Sauerkraut 193

APPENDIX A 195
  Important Micronutrients and Where to Find Them 195
APPENDIX B 202
  Enzymes, Bacteria, and Fibre: The Forgotten Players 202
APPENDIX C 204
  Non-Dairy Sources of Calcium 204
  How Much is Enough? 205
APPENDIX D 206
  Traditional Food Preparation 206
APPENDIX E 208
  Signs and Symptoms of Allergies 208
APPENDIX F 210
  Fatty Acid Deficiency: Detecting and Correcting 210

APPENDIX G	214
How to Do an Elimination Diet	214
Oh My Goodness! What Can I Eat??? Foods To Keep In Stock	216
APPENDIX H	221
Gluten or Gluten-Free?	221
Foods Containing Gluten	223
Nutritional Concerns for the Gluten-Free Diet:	224
Cooking Tips:	224
APPENDIX I	225
Choosing Supplements	225
APPENDIX J	227
Phenols in Food	227
APPENDIX K	229
Common Deficiency Symptoms	229
APPENDIX L	235
Glutamate and Additives	235
APPENDIX M	237
Some Signs of Gut Dysbiosis	237
APPENDIX N	238
Whole Foods to Have Handy	238
REFERENCES	240
ENDNOTES	241
MORE ABOUT THE AUTHOR	255
PERMISSIONS	256
PUBLISHER'S NOTE	257

A Message to the Reader

What I experienced when I had my first child was all too common. After the initial bliss wore off, worry and fear shadowed my days. Feeling overwhelmed somehow became my new norm.

We were living in a quiet log cabin in the woods—a safe haven of sorts—but still, too much of my energy was focused on worry. I worried about chemicals in infant PJs, about car exhaust, that my baby would fall out of bed, or slip out of my hands in the baby bathtub. I was afraid of Sudden Infant Death Syndrome (SIDS), vaccines, illness, pesticides, rashes, and formula. I struggled with breastfeeding, formula caused eczema; we struggled with food intolerance and constipation. I was given conflicting information about supplements and feeding strategies. He was a picky toddler. I wondered if his behaviour and development were normal. I worried about autism.

A primal fear that I would fail to protect my child kept me up at night. I doubted my instincts and didn't know where to turn. The more I learned, the more I worried; the more I wondered if I was a good mother.

My children are older now, and I am at a different stage of parenting. While fear and worry still rise up, I now recognize that they do so when I'm faced with the unknown. Knowledge and experience are the two ingredients that build confidence. When we don't have them, it's so easy to feel powerless, judged, afraid, and confused. We get drawn into panic and obsession on the one hand, or to apathy and defeat on the other. We have to work hard to find a middle ground.

As we grow, our game plan starts to evolve. It expands and changes as we gain insight, and as it does, our confidence increases. Some parenting theories and strategies stick because they resonate, while others get caught by your filter and discarded. If we don't create this filter carefully and consciously, it becomes too easy to be thrown into despair and self-doubt again. An expert interview compels us to throw out groceries and change our menus. A blog article makes us question our style, and a random social media post riddles us with guilt and self-judgment. If you've ever felt this way, I encourage you to work on your filter.

This book is about the food and feeding part of your parenting game plan. It is about what to feed your family, and how to fit healthy food into your busy life. But more importantly, this book will bring you renewed confidence in the role you play in your child's health. I have worked with the most amazing parents over the years who, when they truly embrace their influence, create massive transformation in their children's health. Sleep improves, focus improves, tantrums reduce, learning improves, allergies reduce, growth improves—once parents become active and educated participants in healthcare.

The greatest tool at your disposal is food. The choices you make in the kitchen and grocery store hold profound potential to impact your child's health, but family nutrition is a hard road to navigate and figuring it out can take up an inordinate amount of energy, brain space, and heart. This book will guide you through the clutter and keep you focused. It will give you knowledge and strategies that will instill confidence and help you find a clear path forward.

Let me tell you why you are getting such mixed messages right now about food and health. It's because we are in the midst of a paradigm shift. Over the last ten years or so, revolutionary discoveries have been made about how the body works and how our health is influenced. More details continue to surface and it can be hard to keep up. Just a short time ago, we didn't know that the gut and brain talk to each other via the vagus nerve, that microbes act as metabolic regulators, or that DNA expression can be altered by nutrients and chemicals, and that the digestive tract has its own nervous system. We weren't aware of the intense health effects of inflammation and immune dysregulation, or how those processes can be influenced by our thoughts, behaviours, and food choices. These radical new discoveries have shed a whole new light on what we thought we used to know. They have blown the "dietary-fat-is-bad" myth out of the water, given us new perspectives on the root causes of mental illness, and allergies, given new insights into aging and brain development, and opened up discussion about artificial sugars, gluten, genetically modified foods, and the Standard American Diet as a whole. But it takes time to flesh out new ideas, and for them to take hold or change behaviours and policy. At this point, we have one foot in the old concepts and one in the new. You and I are caught in the midst of change and are left wondering how best to support our kids.

On the positive side, this paradigm shift actually simplifies things. In my nutrition practice, it has helped me boil everything down into a two-pronged process and three core strategies that I have seen accomplish amazing health improvements in a very short time.

The process I take you through in this book will bring you to a place where confidence is allowed to drive, strategy is the trusted co-pilot, tools are in the back seat, and fear ... is in the trunk. The key is to focus on resilience.

Resilience: "The ability to adapt to stress and adversity; the ability of something to return to its original shape after it has been pulled, stretched, pressed, bent, etc.; the ability to become strong, healthy, or successful again after something bad happens." (Merriam-Webster.com 2016)

This is what I want for children; for your children, for mine, for all children; maximal ability to self-regulate when confronted with change, adversity, infection, or turbulence. Regardless of the particular challenges or abilities, the family situations or personalities, strong resilience allows children to become the best version of themselves. This book outlines some very practical strategies, based on solid scientific research and my years of professional practice, which actively support the development of that resilience.

Raising Resilience is about hope, simplicity, and action. It combines my ongoing efforts as a mother with my work as a paediatric nutritionist. *Raising Resilience* will help you understand your child's body and unique needs, recognize indicators when those needs are not being met, and access tools to support them. It will take the focus away from current nutrition dogma and keep your eye on what's most important, so you can relax about the headlines and achieve your health goals without losing your mind in the process. You'll be able to forget about what the rest of the seven billion folks are doing, about the latest trend in Japan, and the latest superfood that you can't get your kids to eat. You'll be able to read a blog post with curiosity rather than self-judgement, deciding with confidence what advice you are willing to let through your filter. You'll be able to ask the right questions of your health care teams and confidently explain your decisions. You will take your rightful place as an active collaborator in your child's wellbeing and growth. You will spend your limited time and energy learning to tune in to your child's body and understand his/her unique and dynamic needs.

Whether you simply want to finally gain some clarity and assurance about your food and feeding strategy, or your child is struggling with a particular problem you want to find a solution to, the plan laid out in this book will help you help your kids become healthier and stronger and will give you renewed confidence in your parenting. I'm excited to dive into this with you.

Acknowledgments

Though the concept of this book started in my head, it blossomed only because of those who supported me along the way.

Thank you to my mother for her unwavering support for everything I do, and her belief in who I am, and to my father for his keen editorial eye, endless support, and enthusiasm.

Thank you to Andy for daring to dream big with me, and to my kids, Benny, Cameron, and Oliver who have been, and continue to be, my greatest teachers.

Thank you to every parent I've ever worked with for inviting me into your life, accepting my support, sharing your struggles and your triumphs. It's your experiences that helped me distill the Raising Resilience system, and it's you who continue to drive me forward; you have taught me more than you could imagine.

Thank you to the unbelievable team at the Ottawa Integrative Health Centre, along with all the health practitioners I've crossed paths with over the years. You inspire me with the work that you do, and you show us all what is possible for children.

Finally, to my wellness business friends and mentors for consistently pushing me out of my own way, and to the fabulous team at I C Publishing for their undying patience and persistence.

Thank you all for helping me to get this book out into the world.

Introduction

The Roots of Resilience

I first became interested in this topic of resilience when I was a high school teacher. I was surprised at the number of young people who were struggling mentally and physically. Recurrent illnesses and infections, aberrant behaviour, learning, mood, and mental health struggles, and sleep conditions, all had become so commonplace that we spent a significant amount of time strategizing about them in teacher meetings. As a team we would assess each student in our small school and troubleshoot their struggles, usually checking for ways to help them find connection, relieve their stress, make them feel safe and empowered, and getting them extra tutoring support.

Many students responded well to our efforts and started to turn around. But some did not, and extreme measures like medication, referrals, or even expulsion became our only recourse. I felt we had failed these kids, and that we were missing something deeper.

I am not anti-medicine, by any means. Diagnoses and medication can offer us a great deal, especially when it comes to crisis intervention. They can be important tools for managing established infection, diffusing suicidal risk, stabilizing mood, or bringing down dangerously high fevers. Diagnoses can be very helpful in getting children extra attention and support. But, as the effect of medication on a child's body continues to be explored and better understood, I become more and more concerned when they are used before all other options have been thoroughly explored.

Raising Resilience

Certain antidepressants have been found to increase aggression and suicidal thoughts in children;[1] antibiotics disrupt our delicate microbiome and can lead to allergy.[2] Even the seemingly innocuous over-the-counter medication acetaminophen has been linked to increased risk of asthma,[3] autism,[4] delayed development,[5] hyperactivity,[6] and liver damage[7] in susceptible individuals. Surely (my teacher-self wondered), while medication can be a fantastic last resort or temporary intervention, there must be more we could do, other avenues we could explore, that could reduce our need for them even further, especially given their potential risks.

It was while working with these students that my interest in the factors which influence a child's natural ability to self-regulate and cope with adversity and expectation was born. I eventually left teaching, and found the answers to my questions and concerns by studying holistic health and nutrition, focusing more specifically on the impact of nutrition and stress on a child's development.

I now work more with parents than with children and, in my nutrition practice, I have seen first-hand how shifting dietary and lifestyle strategies in the ways I outline in this book, helps kids (and their parents for that matter) focus and learn better, relax and sleep well, remain more calm, benefit from reduced infection and allergies, have healthier skin, and enjoy more consistent energy.

Essentially, what I have learned through almost a decade of study and practice is that, given the proper tools and guidance, parents can improve their child's ability to self-regulate and thrive, and reduce their need for medication by boosting the body's innate resources. This is raising resilience.

Let's look at the differences between healthy and reduced resilience, and how we can improve it overall.

Healthy Resilience

The process of raising resilience is based around a simple premise that we have known for centuries and that underlies all types of holistic modalities and medicines; the concept of Homeostasis. Homeostasis is, "the tendency of the body to seek and maintain a condition of balance or equilibrium within its internal environment, even when faced with external changes." (Dictionary.com 2016) We have amazing natural mechanisms that allow us to maintain homeostasis.

For example:
- When it is cold outside our body shunts blood to our vital organs to keep them warm.
- When a virus invades, the immune system sends out patrols to destroy the virus so it can't overcome us.
- When we forget to eat, adrenaline stimulates the release of stored glucose so we don't pass out.
- When we have eaten enough, our satiety hormone, leptin, gets released to tell our brain to stop reaching for food.

The process of achieving homeostasis is actually very dynamic and dozens of feedback mechanisms like these keep us there. We are at our most healthy when these are working well and are not stressed. When we can efficiently maintain homeostasis, we have strong resilience.

Some children, it turns out, are born with these mechanisms intact and strong. These are the children who have great skin, sleep well, learn quickly, and grow healthily; they get over illness quickly and efficiently, respond well to instruction, have a stable weight, good energy, an even temperament, and so on. Their resilience is strong. But asthma, allergies, ADHD, celiac, depression, diabetes, anxiety, paediatric obesity, and autism, are only some of the struggles that are on the rise among children.[8] I see these as signs of reduced resilience.

Raising Resilience

Please allow me to emphasize, I'm not at all proposing that children with these conditions are somehow broken or inadequate. What I am suggesting though, is that these conditions and symptoms are indicators that the body is struggling to achieve homeostasis; that compensatory mechanisms are being overpowered and need support. What I do with my clients, something quickly becoming known as Functional Nutrition, is seek to identify the processes that are struggling, and actively support them by finding a compatible diet strategy. We will delve much deeper into how this works throughout this book.

First, how can diet improve resilience?

Many factors impact resilience. A lot has been written about raising resilience within a social context: how to help our kids make decisions and positive choices, feel grounded and safe, and resolve conflicts, helping them self-regulate as social beings. That is critical information for parents to pull into their strategy, and I do make reference to some of what I consider to be the best resources on that subject. But this book adds another dimension to resilience. It is about physical resilience as well: the body's ability to rebound into a state of balance after it is bent out of shape; addressing what interferes with that ability and how parents can best support it.

Consider this:
- When an anxious moment explodes into a full blown panic attack, despite belly breathing and mental mind tricks, *something else is going on*.
- When simple coughs and colds repeatedly develop into infection requiring antibiotics, despite your diligent use of elderberry and Echinacea, or even medication, *something else is going on*.
- When a child's inability to concentrate and retain what is being taught at school overwhelms a teacher's creative efforts to accommodate, there is *something else going on*.
- When a toddler descends into a fit of rage and aggression when they have to leave a play date, there is *something else going on*.

Introduction • The Roots of Resilience

That "something else" might include the language we use, the connections we establish with our kids, the way we organize our day, all the things your psychologist or family therapist might suggest. But *Raising Resilience* looks at the other dimension I mentioned. It explores some of the underlying *biological* factors that can interfere with all efforts to coach or teach or soothe, and the steps we can take to support our body's natural wisdom and balance—not with medication, but with changes in diet.

No medical condition or behaviour pattern diminishes a child's worth, nor does it reduce our deep love for them. I do believe we need to see, love, and understand our children as they are. But I also believe that every child deserves to live without struggling to breath or focus, without being fearful of certain foods, feeling depressed, anxious, or in pain.

Asking parents to put their five-year-old on Prozac for anxiety, to teach their eight-year-old that certain foods can kill her, to explain to a child that he'll need to take a steroid puffer to every soccer practice, or that he'll need antihistamines for the rest of his life, is not a sufficient solution in my mind. Yet that has become the new normal. That we see more and more children struggling to breathe, focus, move, or function with each generation distresses me profoundly, and I take this trend as a call to action; a call to rally behind the health of all children and offer parents better solutions.

Success Stories

Here are a couple of success stories from my practice in which we used the very same concepts and strategies I present in this book to raise overall resilience, reduce symptoms, and improve health.

Manny:

Dana first contacted me because her four-year-old daughter, Manny, had so many food sensitivities she didn't know what to feed her anymore. Manny had a history of reflux, thrush, and had been on four courses of antibiotics over that year for both ear and urinary tract infections. She was also starting to show signs of what they suspected to be a dust allergy.

To improve Manny's resilience, I first helped Dana find food alternatives so we could reduce inflammation by removing the foods that were irritating her. We used targeted supplements along with some mild fermented foods, antifungal and nutrient-rich teas, antioxidant-rich foods, and fibre to flood her body with nutrients supportive of her digestive system, immune system, and her microbiome.[9] We found gentler yet effective alternatives to the antibiotics which allowed for her bacteria to rebalance.

After two more well-managed infections over the next three months, the infections stopped developing. Over the course of the next year, her reaction to dust subsided, her digestion improved, and we were able to reintroduce many of the foods which used to cause her pain, congestion, and constipation. Her resilience was improving.

Dana and I continued to work together until we had diversified the diet as much as we could, and had devised a nutrient-dense dietary strategy that Dana could stick with. As a result, she felt confident in her ability to understand and meet her daughter's food needs going forward and Manny became a happier, healthier child.

Maggie:

Maggie, age seven, was having panic attacks and bouts of aggression at school, and was about to start the assessment process for ADHD. Her doctor suggested Prozac for the outbursts, but her mother wanted to try non-medical options first. Working alongside the school psychologist and teacher, the family asked me to help them figure out if there were any nutrition-related factors influencing Maggie's behaviours.

We relieved Maggie's chronic constipation by supporting her digestive function with food and supplements. We balanced her blood sugar by focusing on fibre, low glycemic carbohydrates, along with protein-rich breakfasts and snacks, and used small doses of the amino acids, glutamine and GABA. This improved her attention and anxiety, but the behaviours were still concerning.

We discovered and removed some foods to which Maggie was sensitive, and improved the overall nutrient density of the diet, focusing on optimizing proper hormone production and neurological function. Specific supplements including B vitamins, fish oil, and zinc were also incorporated.

At the same time, the teachers experimented with different teaching strategies for Maggie, and the psychologist worked with her on stress management techniques, organization tools, and continued to assess her.

After three months, the teachers reported improved attention and focus; Maggie was sleeping better, and was able to diffuse her panic attacks using breathing techniques. The aggressive outbursts stopped; she was never diagnosed with ADHD and Prozac was never needed. Maggie's case speaks to the effectiveness of this kind of team approach in dealing with learning and behaviour problems noticed at school, without use of medication.

In both these example cases, emerging research on how food influences the body helped us find a starting point. I knew, for example, that chronic constipation can irritate the nervous system, that chronic urinary tract infections can be related to imbalances in gut microflora, that certain critical nutrient deficiencies can hamper the immune system, and that blood sugar instability can trigger anxiety and aggression. From there, because everyone's body is so unique, we needed to engage in a lot of trial and error in order to find a plan that worked.

This process might sound daunting and complicated, but don't panic. The landscape is not as confusing as it might seem at first. If

Raising Resilience

we look a little closer at what seems like an unbelievably complex maze, we find some basic underlying principles. In *Raising Resilience* I will explain these to you and walk you through the process I used with these families so you can apply it, step by step, to your own situation.

How to Use This Book

While our collective understanding of how food and physiology intersect is still evolving, my research and practice has brought me to this simple formula to help parents understand how they can support resilience. It is the formula I use with my clients to explain their health and behaviour concerns, and it helps us remain focused on what's essential to address as we move forward and co-create a plan of action. Here's the formula:

Increased Stress + Decreased Nutrition ⟶ Reduced Resilience

Put another way,

Decreased Stress + Improved Nutrition ⟶ Improved Resilience

This might seem like an oversimplification. And it is, a little. But simplicity is the point. I want you to have it all. I want you to live your wildly creative and inspired life vibrantly and courageously, with confidence and energy while also raising healthy kids and feeling great about your parenting. Too many of us are bogged down, spending way too much time reading and sifting through information without recognizing the inordinate amount of energy it takes, until we hit rock bottom and have nothing left to give. Caring for our children before ourselves is instinctual. If the oxygen masks fall, we will secure our child's first, regardless of instructions. Right? There's no messing with instinct.

That said, it is possible to raise healthy, resilient kids while keeping your own sanity intact; yes it is. However, in order to do that, you need to become spectacularly efficient. You need simple strategies for making quick and effective choices so you can free up the energy you are spending worrying and wondering. What I want you to understand is why the convergence of these two factors—increased stress and decreased nutrition—is playing out so significantly in our kids and how it leads us to a two-step process for improving resilience. You guessed it: decrease stress and increase nutrition.

Step One of the process is to identify and relieve stressors that can throw a body out of balance.

In Part One of *Raising Resilience*, we review the most common stressors that reduce a child's resilience, and I offer suggestions on how to identify and relieve them so you can make room for positive momentum. I also introduce a new perspective to the discussion of stressed-out kids by drawing your attention to common biological factors that are often missed in this debate.

Step Two for raising resilience involves maximizing the tools you have at your disposal to help the body maintain homeostasis and actively support its natural instinct to grow. We do this by focusing in on the three core strategies that are thoroughly explored in Part Two.

Steps One and Two are foundational for raising resilience and, by following them, many symptoms disappear as the body's ability to self-regulate is enhanced. But no book about resilience or family nutrition would be complete though without a section about the impact our relationship with food has on our health.

How we eat, how we talk about food, and how we structure our eating has as deep an impact on our children's health and resilience. Food environment and food relationship is explored in Part Three, along with some very practical suggestions for those of you struggling with picky eaters.

Lastly we discuss transitioning your habits. None of us are superhuman, and we need to find a realistic road forward that works for our families. In Part Four, you'll be introduced to the all-important

HOW TO USE THIS BOOK

80/20 concept. This will help you take a balanced approach as you make changes, and give you an action plan for implementation.

As well, there is a section of appendices at the back of the book. These checklists and charts are there to help you dig deeper into understanding your child's nutritional needs so you can work with your health care teams to develop a strategy that caters to his or her uniqueness.

For change to happen, you need bite-sized, doable strategies, and easy-to-remember instructions. For that reason, you'll find a general summary of the need-to-know elements at the beginning of each section. If you're limited on time and energy, read each summary, and then skip to the strategies and start to implement them.

For those of you who want to sink your teeth into more detail and really understand the why behind the what, you'll find that in the body of each chapter. Gauge for yourself how much you want or need and make your way through *Raising Resilience* accordingly.

By the end of this book, you will have all the tools you need to make some very meaningful modifications to your feeding strategy and will be primed to start seeing some serious health changes in yourself and your family. Will your search for optimal health end here? Likely not. Might you sometimes need outside help, medication, herbs, tinctures, and other therapies? Possibly. But diet is a tool you can learn to use yourself, at home. Looking at what, how, and when you feed your family is one of the best ways to help your kids. It helps you stack the cards in their favour so they can become the healthiest they can be.

Raising resilience is an ongoing and dynamic process, so I have created an online community to support our work together. It's all fine and good to read and understand concepts, but the magic happens when you are able to bring them to life in your kitchen with delicious, nutrient-dense, simple recipes. For some of my favourite food ideas and menus that pull together all the *Raising Resilience* concepts and strategies, check out the Recipes for Resilience section for sample recipes starting on page 129, and find more on my website at JessSherman.com.

Because you are reading this book, I know you have made your child's health a priority. You are developing your game plan and have decided nutrition is important. You are taking time to learn what you need to know. So stop feeling guilty. Take a deep breath. And let's get started raising resilience together so you and your kids can relax, learn, and grow.

PART ONE

UNDERSTANDING DIMINISHED RESILIENCE

Section Overview

In this section, we explore the very important first stage of raising resilience: understanding and reducing stressors. Assessing and addressing your child's stressors minimizes roadblocks so that you can move forward more quickly and easily with your health goals.

We'll look at the impact of three types of stress on the body: social, environmental, and biological. In addition, we'll spend some time learning how the stress response is stimulated in our kids and leads to adverse health effects.

The main focus of this section is on biological stressors; physical factors which can diminish resilience by interfering with, burdening, or blunting the body's ability to self-regulate. I outline the most common biological stressors I see in the families I work with—ones I want every parent to become aware of. They are sugar, environmental toxins, yeast overgrowth, food reactions, genetically modified foods, additives, and lack of sleep. You'll see how these physical stressors diminish resilience, and also find instructions on how to determine if they may be interfering with your child's health and resilience.

Removing Roadblocks

Step One for raising resilience is to remove as many counterproductive factors as possible so we can make room for positive momentum. Stressors are those factors that stimulate a release of inflammatory chemicals, burden the body, and undermine its ability to self-regulate when faced with change, adversity, and turbulence. Quite simply, stress is anything that diverts the body's resources and thus gets in the way of growth and learning.

Now, even if you think this section might not apply to you because you feel your child is generally quite well-adjusted and not under stress, please read on. You may be surprised to learn about hidden stressors and stress responses that don't appear as you may expect them to.

Managing stress is something most of us have already been told to do. Maybe you've tried, and it's crept back into your life. Maybe you don't know where to start, or how to slow down your hamster wheel. Perhaps you're seeing your kids beginning to spin on that same wheel.

Increased stress has a profound influence on our health and has been cited as a contributing factor for many health conditions which are on the rise including anxiety, heart disease, diabetes, and depression. Yet stress remains difficult to manage at times. It sneaks up on us and on our kids and it silently yet profoundly exerts its influence. We have watched each generation carry progressively larger stress loads and we have to work harder than ever to actively reduce them. Our difficulty with stress management is in part because we often miss two very important aspects of it. By drawing our attention to these, we will better be able to evaluate and manage the stress our kids may be under.

The first aspect often missed has to do with how we identify stressors. Most of the conversation we hear about stress management typically focuses on only two out of three types of stressors, the social

PART ONE: Understanding Diminished Resilience

and environmental types. Our kids are too busy, they have too many electronic devices, they are rushed, they experience trauma, or bullying, etc. These are important stressors that certainly do have an impact on resilience. But the third type of contributor to our stress load is often missed. These I am calling biological stressors. Hormone-disrupting chemicals, metals and additives, food sensitivities, sugar, and lack of sleep are examples of some key biological stressors. We'll expand on this much more shortly, specifically learning how to determine if they are interfering with your child's resilience.

The second aspect we tend to miss has to do with the tools we use for stress management. Many of us have been told to exercise, or learn deep breathing, do yoga, or take time for reflection. Therapists work with children to express themselves or learn coping skills. Yes, those strategies can be very helpful, and I'm completely in favour of using them to help our kids because they actively create positive physiological changes in the body. Deep breathing and meditation have been shown to reduce cortisol levels, and yoga and mindful meditation can help stimulate calming neurotransmitters, for example.[10]

But here's what we often overlook: reduced physical resilience reduces our ability to tolerate stress. Our body has intricate and fascinating ways of dealing with stress, which you'll read about in this section. When you learn how our stress management system works, you'll see how our physical ability to cope with stressors can become impaired when the body's resilience is low. When this happens, even the smallest trigger can set off the stress response. You'll understand how supporting the players of our body's stress management system improves our ability to handle stress, making us less volatile, less anxious, and more focused. Supporting the health of the liver so it can flush hormones from the body, and ensuring proper nutrition so that neurotransmitters and hormones function and the adrenal glands stay healthy are examples of some of the vital steps for improving our body's ability to cope with the inevitable stressors of life.

Raising Resilience

Have you ever wondered why one person can stay calm, cool, and collected in the face of life's pressures while another will completely lose it and fall apart under the slightest pressure? The way I see it, the person who holds it together has a combination of better management tools and a healthier management system. As you start to identify and remove the stressors we talk about here and begin to implement the three core strategies that support resilience discussed in Part Two, you will find that not only does your child have less stress to cope with, but they also enjoy an improved ability to handle stress because you have more tools to help strengthen their stress management system.

Understanding Stress

See if any of these situations ring a bell:

> You are already five minutes late and your kids can't find their shoes ... your heart starts to beat faster and jumps into your throat.
>
> You stay up late watching reruns for six nights straight and then find you start craving sugar and feel disoriented at work.
>
> Your child binges on Hallowe'en candy and then gets the flu two days later.
>
> You eat a meal and then end up flat on the couch ten minutes later.

These are examples of the body responding to stressors. Something has triggered the initiation of changes in the body, and you experience symptoms as a result. Sometimes the trigger and symptom are obvious, like your slow-poke child triggering your anxiety. Often they are more difficult to determine, like a food sensitivity causing fatigue, or lack of sleep causing sugar cravings.

In this section, we'll look at how and why stressors generate symptoms and how that lowers resilience. From there, we'll discuss how

PART ONE: Understanding Diminished Resilience

to identify stressors your children might be exposed to so you can take steps to relieve them.

First, let's look at classic stress. Stress is typically defined as a state in which the body's fight or flight response is activated. It is a physiological response to an event, the anticipation of an event, or the perception of a situation. The body releases chemicals which result in changes we can often (though not always) feel and see.

We're all familiar, for example, with the sensation of watching our child clamber too high on a rock wall or climbing apparatus at the park. We become stressed because we worry she will fall and hurt herself. In this case, we are responding to the anticipation of an event. A cascade of hormones and neurotransmitters is involved in this response. The pituitary gland, the hypothalamus, and the adrenal glands—collectively known as the Hypothalamus-Pituitary-Adrenal axis (the HPA axis)—are working together to initiate your body's reaction: pounding heart, flushed face, tensed muscles, etc. The stress response is a marvellous feedback mechanism designed to keep you safe and able to deal with crisis, but let's look a little deeper to understand how it can impact resilience.

The stress response is managed by hormones and neurotransmitters which are chemical messengers in our bodies. They travel through the body and orchestrate complex processes, including the stress response. Some are predominantly excitatory, meaning they speed up processes, and others are mostly inhibitory, meaning they tend to slow processes down. Some can do both, depending on the situation. These excitatory and inhibitory chemicals teeter-totter, talking to each other and working together to maintain a dynamic state of balance. Together, they influence every single organ and system of the body.

Adrenaline and cortisol feature prominently in the classic stress response and are the ones most associated with that stressed-out feeling and the subsequent adverse health effects. Both are released by the adrenal glands and have a predominantly excitatory effect. Back to your child climbing on the climber; adrenaline increases your heart rate, shuts down your digestion (i.e. makes you feel sick to your stomach), dilates your pupils, and increases your blood pressure. Cortisol increases your blood sugar so you can quickly run to the rescue should your child fall, and, on a deeper level, it shuts down the production of thyroid hormone and suppresses the immune system which is not needed in the moment.

These chemicals essentially divert your resources from what is not essential in the moment, in order to prioritize your ability to fight, flee, or act quickly. Once your child returns safely to the ground with a huge smile on her face, the production of these excitatory hormones should be shut off and balanced by the inhibitory hormones. Danger has passed (or, in this case, potential danger) and your body's chemistry can return to a calm state.

But sometimes we don't relax. Sometimes, our child returns safely to the ground, yet we continue to play the "what if" game in our heads. We get angry at them, lash out, and insist we're going home—park time is over. Tomorrow's outing is cancelled. We stomp off in a huff, and so on.

When we don't calm down (and there can be a variety of reasons for this), we enter a more chronic stage of stress. Our stress response remains activated. Our adrenal glands have to keep pumping out adrenaline and cortisol, the heart continues to be stimulated to beat faster, the immune system and thyroid continue to be suppressed, and digestion remains shut down, etc., etc. You continue to feel "on edge," jumpy and reactive. You snap and freak out at the littlest thing. That night you have no appetite for dinner and you might feel wired and unable to sleep; all because of the stress hormones. In a moment, we'll look at how this kind of chronic stress can be activated in children. First, though, let's look a little deeper into the downstream health effects of this kind of chronic stress.

PART ONE: Understanding Diminished Resilience

Because it interferes with our hormonal balance and because, you'll remember, hormones and neurotransmitters influence every system of the body, stress has been associated with just about every condition and disease state. Depression, hypothyroidism, acne, PMS, constipation, aggression, fatigue, insomnia, headaches, anxiety, infertility, hyperactivity, and sleep troubles can all be linked, in part, to hormonal and neurotransmitter imbalance which can be triggered by stress. Inflammation, immune dysregulation and digestive imbalances, which have in turn been connected to autistic symptoms, ADHD, allergy, anxiety and depression, heart disease, Alzheimer's, and diabetes, can also be attributed in part to dysregulated stress hormones, most notably cortisol. Recent research on the developing brain tells us that when an infant or child is exposed to prolonged activation of the stress response, their neural pathways are actually altered, placing them at higher risk for heart disease, diabetes, depression, and substance abuse down the road.[11]

Stress-induced hormone imbalance is a game-changer when it comes to our health. Even if we are eating well, exercising, doing everything we're advised, an inability to self-stabilize the hormonal teeter-totter will undermine our efforts because of the strong physiological effects. In this way, stress acts as a barrier to resilience, interfering with what our kids are supposed to be doing, which is learning and growing.

How do we mitigate the damage caused by stress? As mentioned, there are two ways: reduce stressors, and strengthen our body's stress response. You'll learn how to strengthen the body's stress response with good nutrition in Part Two; below, you'll learn how to find and reduce some common stressors to which our kids are exposed.

QUICK NOTE: Cortisol Concerns

The only way to know for sure if cortisol imbalance is a problem for your child is to have your doctor do a test. Saliva or hair analysis tests are more helpful than blood tests because they show not only a snapshot of cortisol levels but a pattern of dips and spikes over time.

Here are a few symptoms which might indicate cortisol levels or patterns are less than optimal:
- Overly stressed, anxious, depressed, overactive, or overwhelmed
- Freaks out when something unplanned occurs
- Intense sugar cravings
- Feels easily tired, but has trouble falling asleep or staying asleep
- Can't get out of bed in the morning
- Has to pee frequently in the middle of the night (beyond what is normal child development)
- Has headaches
- Catches every cold going around and doesn't kick it quickly, takes a long time to heal from scrapes and cuts
- Feels quite light-headed or faint when they move quickly from lying to standing
- If your child has been diagnosed with sub-optimal thyroid hormones, it could be that cortisol is at play because it shuts down the production of these hormones

If your child is dealing with three or more of these issues, look closely at their stressors in an effort to control cortisol. If this doesn't help, see your doctor about doing some tests.

QUICK NOTE
Your child's hyperactivity, inability to focus, or her lethargy and fatigue might be caused in part by a hormone/neurotransmitter imbalance. Excitatory chemicals associated with the stress response such as adrenaline, norepinephrine, and cortisol are meant to live in balance with the predominantly inhibitory chemicals like GABA and serotonin. But a dominance of excitatory chemicals keeps the body in a tense state and inhibits its ability to rest, digest, and grow. On the flip side, a dominance of calming chemicals can result in feelings of apathy, fatigue, and lack of focus; this is equally as problematic for

PART ONE: Understanding Diminished Resilience

our kids. If you are struggling with this, pay particular attention to identifying and reducing their stressors and talk to your health care team about amino acids and nutrients that can help stabilize the hormonal balance.

Identifying and Reducing Stressors in Children

A certain amount of short-term stress is not a problem. We have mechanisms to deal with it, and experiencing some can even be quite beneficial to growth and development. It's ongoing, chronic stress—the type we're not able to turn off—which is the kind we want to reduce.

Ascertaining chronic stressors in adults can be straightforward: job, marriage, money, etc. What worries a child, though? I mentioned three sources of stressors. The two main potential sources of stress that can reduce resilience by continually stimulating the HPA axis are the social and environmental sources. We'll touch on them briefly before turning to the third category, biological stressors, which can also throw the body into hormonal disequilibrium, though in a slightly different manner.

Social Stress

This category includes all issues of relationship. We are creatures of attachment and need strong social supports to feel confident and secure. We also need a strong sense of purpose, identity, and belonging. By instinct, children look to others to learn how they are supposed to move in the world. When they feel unsure or insecure, children can also feel disoriented. This can be a major source of stress, reducing their productivity, confidence, and overall health.[12]

Helping a child to manage social stress and creating circumstances and environments that help them feel secure is another book topic entirely. But now that you understand how the stress response works, you can start to connect the dots and understand how feelings of insecurity, abandonment, lack of attachment, and lack of purpose can reduce resilience by stimulating stress hormones.

For further guidance on finding strategies for identifying and relieving social stress, I suggest you look to child and family therapists, BodyTalk™ workers, or psychotherapists who understand the role of attachment in parenting. You'll discover some of my favourite resources discussed on my website.

To recognize possible social stressors, consider your child's relationship with
- parents
- siblings
- caregivers
- peers
- teachers
- coaches
- extended family
- friends

Try looking through the eyes of your child for relationships that might evoke feelings of emotional instability, fear, overstimulation, and being overwhelmed. As well, look for the absence of strong connections in your child's life. These can point you to sources of social stress for them.

> **QUICK NOTE**
> Simple strategies recommended for relieving social stress:
> - Create a predictable routine for your child.
> - Get suitable support for your child if he/she has experienced trauma.
> - Foster strong, healthy attachments between your child and adults in the community beyond the parents.
> - Communicate clearly and often with your child's teachers.
> - Get to know your child's friends.
> - Find time to connect deeply with your child, engaging in

PART ONE: Understanding Diminished Resilience

shared experiences.
- Involve your child in community initiatives.
- Encourage them to get involved in school initiatives (if age appropriate).
- Involve your child in a sport or club (or do this with your child).

Creating strong and meaningful connections between your child and yourself, between your child and your community, and aiding in tapping into his inner resources can help stabilize and ground a child. This can relieve their stress, reduce circulating stress hormones, improve confidence, promote self-actualization, and resilience.

Environmental Stress

This category refers to stress generated by your child's environment. Some children's stress response gets activated by too much clutter, too many choices, brash colours, over-scheduling, and harsh sounds, all of which can overpower them and add to circulating stress hormones.

Also included here would be the stress generated by electromagnetic radiation from cellular phone towers, cordless phones, smart meters, Wi-Fi, and cell phones. A great deal has been written about the possible impact of electromagnetic stress, particularly on the growing body and brain, though we need to know more about it. In 2013, Martha Herbert, a paediatric neurologist and leader in autism research at Harvard Medical School, compiled over 550 citations that document the adverse health and neurological impact of electromagnetic radiation, particularly influencing the brains of children and older adults.[13]

It's not well understood whether electromagnetic radiation is actually causing reduced resilience, or if it only becomes an issue once resilience is diminished by other means. Regardless, it is worth considering the amount your child is exposed to this environmental stressor, particularly if they are struggling.

> **QUICK NOTE**
> Some strategies to reduce environmental stressors:
> - Choose soothing colours for the walls of your home and your child's bedroom.
> - Avoid cluttering a child's play space and bedroom with too many toys, books, and pictures.
> - Throw out old and broken books and toys.
> - Find or create small cozy spaces that they can make their own.
> - Be aware of the sounds in your home, including loud music and the radio.
> - Be aware of the smells in your home.
> - Avoid over-scheduling.
> - Reduce TV and screen time.
> - Remove Electromagnetic Field sources from your child's bedroom, limit cell phone and cordless phone use.

As with the social stressors, managing environmental stressors will help support resilience by calming the stress response.

Biological Stress

Biological stressors are the ones I spend most of my energy addressing with my clients. As mentioned, they often go unnoticed but can pose a major roadblock when you are trying to improve your child's health.

Biological stress refers to the physiological changes in the body caused by things like food intolerance, yeast overgrowth, gut dysbiosis, sugar, and additives. It also includes stress caused by ingested, inhaled, and absorbed chemicals and metals like BPA, lead, arsenic, and organophosphates. These stressors result in the same kind of hormonal disequilibrium as classic stress and generally cause increased work for the body.

PART ONE: Understanding Diminished Resilience

I've outlined some of the most common biological stressors that interfere with resilience in children, to describe here. Certainly, there are others. You might hear of health conditions reversing after eradicating hidden underlying infections, parasites, or moulds, or after correcting eye sight or spinal alignment. You might read how things like caesarean, tobacco smoke, and certain medications can be stressors which adversely affect our resilience and increase our risk of illness.[14]

All of this is worthy of consideration as you develop your family's health plan. However, as a nutritionist, I consider the stressors listed here as fundamental. They are largely within your ability to manage and their influence on health is well documented. Relieving them will give you a big bang for your buck. Don't panic over them; just become aware that they can act as barriers and might require some extra attention. As you implement the three core strategies in Part Two of this book, some of these stressors will naturally resolve.

Top Biological Stressors
Sugar
The average American eats about 165 lb. of added sugar each year.[15] That doesn't even include the naturally occurring sugar in carbohydrate-rich food. The American Heart Association suggests added sugar should be no more than 6 tsp a day for women and 9 tsp a day for men.[16] That would make it about 3 to 4 tsp a day for a child. The average is between 20 to 33 tsp of added sugar daily.

The glucose that we get from sugar is an essential nutrient that we use to create energy, but there are several ways excessive dietary sugar interferes with resilience.

The first has to do with sugar's effect on blood sugar. The importance of controlling fluctuating blood sugar is so profound that I devote an entire core principle to it in Part Two. We'll look closely at blood sugar starting on page 87. For now, we'll look at the basic overview of how dietary sugar reduces resilience because of its effect on blood sugar.

Blood glucose levels are regulated by an amazing feedback loop driven by hormones. When we eat sugar or a carbohydrate-rich food, the level of glucose in our blood goes up. Our pancreas responds by releasing insulin which shuttles the sugar into our cells where it is used to make energy. This makes our blood sugar level go back down. When blood sugar falls to a certain level, our hunger hormones kick in and we reach for more food to increase it again. If we don't get that food in, the adrenal glands and liver come to the rescue, stimulating the release of stored glucose so we don't pass out.

When we eat too much sugar (or for that matter, not enough) we place stress on this feedback system. The pancreas, adrenal glands, and liver feel the impact directly, and the brain, the thyroid, immune system, and digestion, all feel the impact by extension. Because of the hormones involved in blood sugar management, (you'll recall that hormones influence every system of the body), symptoms of fluctuating blood sugar can be diverse. Lethargy, fatigue, depression, nervousness, poor memory, difficulty concentrating, dizziness, insomnia, frequent infections, weight gain, panic attacks, and anxiety are all symptoms that can be helped by stabilizing blood sugar. Wide sugar fluctuations can also lead to weight gain, obesity, and type 2 diabetes, which in turn are risk factors for cardiovascular disease, Alzheimer's, and cancer.[17]

There is a second, less obvious, though still important way sugar is an obstacle to resilience, and it has to do with its effect on vitamins and minerals. High sugar intake and high insulin levels have been shown to decrease levels of vitamin C, magnesium, calcium, and chromium either by increasing requirements, stimulating excretion, or decreasing absorption.[18] These essential micronutrients help control heart rhythm, vascular tone, nerve function, bone formation,

PART ONE: Understanding Diminished Resilience

immune function, cellular stability, muscle contraction, and relaxation and, not so surprisingly, carbohydrate metabolism.

Magnesium and chromium are particularly interesting because they help regulate blood sugar directly. So, in a vicious cycle sort of way, sugar depletes these minerals and then the low levels reduce our ability to manage sugar and increase our risk for type 2 diabetes and related diseases.[19]

And yes, there's more. Sugar has also been found to disturb white blood cell function (i.e. decrease immune function), disrupt metabolic hormones, slow digestive function, feed pathogenic gut bacteria, and cause low grade inflammation and oxidative stress (we'll expand on oxidative stress later).[20]

Now don't get me wrong. A little candy here and there is not a reason to panic (we'll talk about finding balance in Part Four), but you can see now how dietary sugar puts a lot of stress on our body and interferes with our goal of raising resilience. Sugar has an immediate impact on mood and function and also has a long-term impact on overall health and risk for disease. Excessive sugar causes problems. Plain and simple. We'll delve much more deeply into sugar and strategies for managing it in Part Two.

QUICK NOTE: Not all sugar is called "sugar" on food labels.

Here are some other names for sugar to look out for at the grocery store:
- corn syrup
- corn syrup solids
- high fructose corn syrup
- glucose-fructose
- fructose
- dextrose
- maltose
- malt

- maltodextrin
- invert sugar
- ingredients that end in "ose" (sucrose, glucose, etc.)
- ingredients that end in "ol" (mannitol, xylitol, maltitol, etc.)
- evaporated cane juice
- sorghum syrup
- turbinado
- malt syrup
- Sucanat
- rapadura
- molasses
- honey
- palm sugar or coconut sugar
- maple syrup
- brown rice syrup

QUICK NOTE:

Does your child show any of these symptoms? Stabilizing blood sugar as described in Part Two can help.

- sleeplessness
- temper tantrums
- crying for no apparent reason
- hyperactive/overactive
- uncontrollable
- angry/hostile
- distractible
- Jekyll/Hyde behaviour
- headaches
- moody, depressed, anxious
- can't sit still
- shaky/irritable before or after meals
- agitation
- defiance
- exhausted after meals
- cravings for carbohydrates or sugar

PART ONE: Understanding Diminished Resilience

Environmental Toxins

Pesticides, metals, fragrances, additives; toxins are everywhere. They are in the air we breathe, the food we eat, our clothes and bedding, creams, and bubble-bath, cleaners, toothpaste—everywhere. Like sugar, they reduce resilience because our body has to spend precious energy and resources dealing with them.

Here's an example of how toxins from our food and environment can impact our resilience. Recently, researchers at the Massachusetts Institute of Technology (MIT), have been studying glyphosate, the main industrial chemical in agriculture, and particularly looking at its impact on the body. So far, some of their findings suggest that it might make the pineal gland susceptible to aluminium toxicity, reduce sulphur, glutathione, and magnesium in the body, impair phase one liver detoxification enzymes, impair vitamin D synthesis, and actively destroy gut bacteria.[21] According to these researchers, pesticides, including glyphosate, have the potential of disabling the on/off switch of the immune system, leading to a state of hyperactive immune stimulation.[22] So, these chemicals could be having a detrimental impact on our hormonal and detoxification systems and, as a result, our resilience. In 2015, seventeen experts from eleven countries labelled glyphosate as "a probable human carcinogen."[23] The MIT investigation gives us a possible explanation for its cancer-causing effect.

Other chemicals, like BPA, found in cans and plastics, phthalates found in plastic wrap, toys, and some cosmetics, and organophosphate pesticides, are known to disrupt our hormone creation and signalling, further reducing resilience.[24]

Luckily, our bodies are equipped with an amazing detoxification system—the complexity of which we are still uncovering—and we can deal with a certain level of toxicity. We do one of three things when we inhale, inject, or absorb a toxin from our environment or food: we neutralize and flush it with the help of the gut bacteria, the liver, enzymes, and nutrients; our immune system attacks and destroys it; or we tuck it away, usually in fat cells.

However, it's important to realise that regardless of whether a certain chemical or metal has been approved as safe, or safe levels have been established, when a foreign substance is introduced into the body, the body has to deal with it. "Safe" only means that we have a mechanism for dealing with it. The question remains: can our bodies keep up with the ever increasing amount to which it is exposed daily?

Many think not. Consider the conclusions of these researchers concerning the impact of toxins on brain function:

> "We postulate that modern day environmental toxicant exposure, along with major changes in our food supply and lifestyle practices, has had a profound impact on the body's ability to absorb and utilize nutrients critical for brain health. Furthermore, we propose that these factors are markedly altering the body's natural state such that neuro-critical nutrients are so depleted and/or functionally deficient that the normal processes of homeostatic balance and resilience are no longer functional." (Wendy A. Morley and Stephanie Seneff 2014)

They found that environmental toxins inhibit the absorption of critical nutrients we need to function, and this forces our bodies to compensate. In other words, environmental toxins reduce our resilience.

Metals and chemicals in our environment and food represent a physical stress on the body and contribute to diminished resilience on two fronts: first, their very presence requires an increased amount of nutrients and enzymes to flush them from the body, and our organs responsible for detoxification are given an increased work load; second, they can interfere with organ function by depleting nutrients, blocking receptor sites, creating oxidative stress and inflammation, and interfere with biochemical processes. They may also interfere with mitochondria function, the energy powerhouse of the body.[25]

The best case scenario when it comes to environmental toxins is that your child's body is well equipped to detoxify; they inherited a relatively low toxic burden and a high nutrient status, and thus they have some good reserve and won't feel the effects of chemical toxicity until later in life. Worst case scenario is that environmental chemicals overcome the body's ability to cope with them and have an immediate impact on brain development and growth. Either way, these chemicals and metals represent a barrier to resilience as they are a burden to the body.

QUICK NOTE

Is toxicity an issue for your child? We are learning that some children have reduced detoxification capabilities than others due to a host of factors including genetic make-up, nutrient deficiencies, and a high toxic load at birth.[26] Does your child have trouble concentrating? Have skin conditions? Have inconsistent energy? A sluggish immune system? Mood swings? Slow wound healing? Tics? If so, reducing this stressor can help. Switch to safer cleaning products and personal care products, switch plastic food storage containers and water bottles to stainless or glass, consider the air quality in your home and car (test for mould, avoid air fresheners), read food labels carefully and find clean sources of food. Cleaning up the diet and the home is an important way to reduce this stressor. Also talk with your healthcare teams about improving your child's detoxification processes.

Further, researchers are finding that improving nutritional status can become a key tool to improve detoxification.[27] More on this in Part Two.

Genetically Modified Foods (GMs or GMOs)

Third party researchers (those not involved in the GM industry) have raised at least sixty concerns that reflect the need for further research on genetically modified foods and the chemicals associated with them.[28]

More and more doctors are finding that having their patients avoid genetically modified foods has helped relieve symptoms of asthma, allergies, arthritis, and more. In 2009, the American Society of Environmental Medicine called for a complete moratorium on GM foods due to the health effects they were noticing in clinical practice.[29]

We don't know exactly why or how genetically modified food affects resilience. Perhaps it is the food itself, or the increase of chemicals used in its production, or the sheer quantity of it to which we are exposed via animal feed and additives.[30] But the potential dangers, which include increased risk of allergy, reduced fertility, and the complete hijacking of the immune system, are so severe that we need to find out.

We need more details about this and further research on the possible effects of GM foods on the body. Until that happens, I caution parents who are trying to boost resilience, to avoid them when possible. Visit www.nongmoproject.org to download a complete list and shopping guide to help you avoid GMOs, and visit my website to stay up-to-date with emerging research.

Candida Yeast

A yeast called Candida Albicans is naturally present in all of us. While it is naturally found in the body's internal ecosystem, it's usually held in check by probiotic (or beneficial) bacteria.

Candida can become a problem when certain circumstances that suppress probiotic bacteria such as sugar, chlorine, stress, antibiotics, and some medications create an environment in which it can multiply and get out of control. When candida gets out of control, an infection called candidiasis can develop. If this happens, the yeast can generate chemicals that interfere with function. Acetaldehyde, carbon monoxide, arabinose, and other compounds created in the digestive tract when yeast is abundant can cross the digestive barrier and interfere with the proper functioning of the body in a variety of ways. Acetaldehyde, for example, directly suppresses T-cells of the immune system and is classified as a class 1 carcinogen,[31] and arabinose might cause a deficiency in B vitamins as well as leaky gut. There are about eighty known toxic compounds potentially secreted by candida yeast,[32] many of which can effect growth, ability to learn, and behaviour.

A child could develop a yeast imbalance because it crossed the placenta,[33] or was picked up in the birth canal during birth. Perhaps they needed a round of antibiotics or other medication which created an opportunity for yeast to proliferate. Yeast also thrive when the diet is high in sugar. The stress hormone cortisol, has an adverse effect on beneficial gut bacteria, so chronic stress can increase the likelihood for candida to thrive.

QUICK NOTE
Classic indicators of yeast overgrowth:
- foggy thinking
- irrational behaviour
- impulsivity
- fatigue
- spaciness
- aggression
- itchy, dry skin
- hypersensitivity
- diaper rash
- recurrent infections
- cravings for sweets
- giggle fits
- sleep disturbances
- perseverative (repetitive behaviour)[34]

Raising Resilience

We will discuss much more about ways to keep candida yeast from becoming a problem in the digestion section in Part Two.

At this point, I simply want you to understand that candida can reduce resilience because it is one of several pathogenic microbes which create chemicals in the body that circulate in the blood and interfere with proper function. There are other pathogenic yeasts and bacteria that do this too; here I highlight this particular yeast as it seems to be the most common. Review the previous QUICK NOTE to determine if yeast overgrowth might be a factor driving your child's troubling symptoms or behaviours. It can be quite a relief to understand that your child's behaviour is actually driven by something other than her desire to push your buttons!

If your child already has a yeast overgrowth, you'll need to work with a practitioner to actively pull that yeast back to acceptable levels and reorganize the gut microbiome. You'll learn proactive steps to take in Part Two to make sure it remains held in check.

Adverse Food Reactions

Back in the early 1900s, the definition of an allergy was any type of altered reaction to a common substance. The term was used to explain why one person starts sneezing in response to pollen while another person doesn't, for example. In the late 1960s, shortly after it was discovered that the immune system had various types of workers (called immunoglobulins), the definition was narrowed to include only adverse reactions caused specifically by activation of a particular immunoglobulin, the immunoglobulin E (or IgE). That definition still largely dominates conventional thought on allergies today, and your typical allergy test looks only for the presence of IgE antibodies for diagnosis.

When an allergy-like reaction is observed, but testing reveals no IgE, the condition is often called a sensitivity. The mechanism of these reactions is complex and not fully understood; however, it

PART ONE: Understanding Diminished Resilience

involves the release of inflammatory chemicals called cytokines and prostaglandins as a result of the stimulation of other types of immunoglobulins, including IgG and IgA.

There is a third category of food reaction which can provoke equally as profound symptoms, but does not involve the immune system at all. Lactose intolerance, for example, is a food reaction caused by the lack of a certain enzyme that digests milk sugar. Various chemicals in foods like glutamate, salicylates, and amines can cause allergy-like symptoms by irritating nerve endings around the body. We'll talk more about these chemicals when we talk about additives.

Upwards of two hundred different symptoms, ranging from body aches to self-injurious behaviour (as found in autism, for example), and diabetes have been associated with food reactions.[35] Constipation, skin rashes, sleep disturbances, headaches, body aches, fatigue, spaciness, and hyperactivity are some of the more common signs that can indicate food intolerance. A more complete list can be found in Appendix E.

While it can be difficult to identify food reactions, I have seen a wide variety of symptoms reverse relatively quickly after the elimination of offending foods.

Here's how an undiagnosed food reaction presents a barrier to resilience:

- The allergic response triggers inflammatory compounds called prostaglandins which decrease pancreatic function, leaving the body at risk for enzyme depletion (and resulting nutrient depletion) and hypoglycaemia (refer back to the discussion about sugar to remember why hypoglycaemia reduces resilience).
- The symptoms such as spaciness, constipation, depression, skin rashes, fatigue, and hyperactivity interfere with a child's ability to learn and thrive.

- The response leads to gut irritation and a reduced ability to absorb nutrients, ultimately leading to under-nourishment and opening the door to candida overgrowth (refer back to the discussion about candida on pages 46–48).
- Allergy is an immune response, and continual stimulation of the immune system may lead to reduced or altered function of this supremely important protective system.

True allergies are fairly easy to have diagnosed. IgE testing is pretty accurate and can be requested through your primary doctor. But because the list of symptoms associated with intolerance/sensitivity is so vast, and because it can take four or five days for symptoms to manifest after exposure to a trigger, it can be frustrating to try to identify them. Testing for IgG, IgA, and IgM can be expensive but can be ordered by your doctor or nutritionist and be a helpful guide. An elimination-provocation diet is considered the most effective way to identify a food sensitivity/intolerance. You'll find instructions for how to do that in Appendix G.

Food reactions represent a barrier to resilience, and when we cover the gut-allergy connection and digestion in Part Two, we'll elaborate on how to relieve the burden of allergens.

Additives

Additives include any non-food compound that is added to food to produce a technical effect. Fragrances, dyes, preservatives, and stabilizers are some examples. Reference was made to additives when I explained the burden of environmental chemicals, but I bring it back here to discuss a few additives in particular that pose a problem for many children.

Back in the 1970s, researchers started to notice the impact that certain additives had on select children, particularly on hyperactive children.[36] Dr. Ben Feingold created the Feingold Diet which focused

PART ONE: Understanding Diminished Resilience

on removing additives, colouring, and natural salicylates, arguing that this diet improved learning, behaviour, and function in his study group. Over the next few decades, his theories were largely dismissed as anecdotal and the result of a placebo effect, as his studies could not be replicated.[37] Yet, many families continue to experience the Feingold effect and doctors who have seen similar results continue to defend his findings.[38]

I have encountered some children who react directly to additives and do better when these additives are removed. We now understand these reactions to involve nerve stimulation as described above. They are also associated with a lack of certain nutrients and enzymes. For example, reactions to glutamate-based additives like MSG, including headaches and hyperactivity, have been linked to B6 deficiency and low levels of glutathione.[39] Reactions to phenol-based additives have been linked to zinc and fatty acid deficits, along with certain enzyme deficiencies. These hyper-sensitive children are supported almost immediately by a low additive, nutrient-dense diet that removes the irritation and re-establishes their enzymes and nutrients. See the following QUICK NOTES to figure out if these additives are causing a reaction in your child.

Putting a child on an additive-free diet requires that you increase the real food in their diet, ones full of the nutrients that support resilience. This was aptly pointed out in defence of Dr. Feingold in the mid-1980s. Dr. Bernard Rimland, PhD, wrote, ". . . children who have been on the Feingold diet for a time tend to be … more able to withstand the food additive challenge. … the Feingold diet tends to keep the child from consuming sugary, non-nutritious 'junk food.' The child consequently increases his intake of genuine food containing the vitamins, minerals, amino acids, and other nutrients necessary for proper functioning of the brain."[40] Basically, what Dr. Rimland is pointing out, is that when you take out additives, you improve on one of the three core strategies you'll learn about in Part Two, nutrient density. When you do that, a child's resilience is improved and they become less reactive to the chemical stressors found in junk food.

A nutrient-dense, additive-free diet bolsters resilience. It can reduce symptoms interfering with a child's ability to thrive, and it can also restore the proper nutrition that is foundational to resilience. As you clean up the diet and improve overall nutrient density and absorption, as described in the next few sections of this book, your child will be better able to handle occasional exposure to additives, and you will reduce the potential stress and symptoms they can cause.

QUICK NOTE
Classic signs of phenol intolerance:
- hyperactivity
- self-injurious behaviour
- impatience
- headaches
- red cheeks and ears
- aggression
- unusual cravings for phenolic-rich foods (see Appendix J)

Typically, a reaction to phenols happens within two hours of it being ingested, though it can sometimes be delayed up to forty-eight hours. Children with a sensitivity to phenols often lack a particular enzyme needed to metabolize them called phenol-sulfo-transferase. They tend to react strongly to certain food dyes and additives and sometimes, if the intolerance is quite severe, foods that are naturally high in phenols (see Appendix J for a food list).

QUICK NOTE – Glutamate
Glutamate is an amino acid found in many foods. Like phenols, there is nothing inherently bad about glutamate; in fact, it is essential for health. However, in children who cannot process it effectively, it can act as an excitatory neurotransmitter that can stimulate inflammation and lead to hormone imbalance,

particularly insufficient GABA, a calming neurotransmitter. Some symptoms that could be a glutamate reaction include:
- hyperactivity
- anxiety
- sleep troubles
- swelling
- burning
- flushing
- headaches
- heart palpitation
- numbness/tingling in mouth
- excessive sweating
- difficulty calming down
- heightened sensory sensitivity
- aggression
- irritability
- tics
- emotional outbursts

See Appendix L for foods and additives high in glutamate.

Lack of Sleep

In 2016, the American Academy of Sleep Medicine, released the most specific guidelines to date for how much sleep our kids should be getting.[41] Their recommendations are as follows:

4 to 12 month olds:	12 to 16 hours
1 to 2 year olds:	11 to 14 hours
3 to 5 year olds:	10 to 13 hours
6 to 12 year olds:	9 to 12 hours
13 to 18 year olds:	8 to 10 hours

Sleep timing, duration, and quality all influence the organization of our hormones and the function of our nervous system, and as such, inadequate sleep can serve as a major strain on the body and a barrier to resilience. Sleep actually has an impact on every single system of the body. Though she looks calm and peaceful, your child is hard at work when she sleeps.

I'm pretty sure you already know how a bad night's sleep makes you feel. After all, most of us have been through those early days with babies. But like the other biological stressors mentioned here, inadequate sleep has a deep impact on your body's systems. Poor sleep has been shown to influence weight, appetite, and glucose control,[42] can lead to depression,[43] poor tissue repair,[44] reduced memory and ability to learn,[45] and increases the risk of obesity, heart disease, diabetes, high blood pressure, and stroke.[46] Our hunger and satiety hormones, ghrelin and leptin, become dysregulated when we don't sleep enough,[47] so even your child's appetite and eating pattern might be changing because she is not getting enough sleep. Further, production and function of many hormones, including growth, thyroid, and sex hormones require adequate sleep.

Interestingly, cortisol comes into play again here. You'll remember cortisol as one of our major excitatory hormones released by the adrenal glands when our stress response, the HPA axis, is stimulated. Various studies have shown that when a person is chronically sleep deprived, their evening cortisol level is higher by up to six-fold.[48] Cortisol is meant to be low at night, allowing us to slip into sleep with the help of melatonin. In this way, poor sleep begets poor sleep. The HPA axis is overstimulated and the parasympathetic branch of the nervous system, the branch associated with rest and regeneration, is never allowed to function properly. High circulating cortisol can also lead to high blood sugar and all the associated effects we've touched on so far. All in all, this amounts to a major stress on the body triggered by inadequate sleep.

Sleep is an essential time during which the body creates and resets hormones, detoxifies, and integrates knowledge. We are meant to live within a sleep-wake rhythm that follows daylight patterns, called

PART ONE: Understanding Diminished Resilience

the circadian rhythm. When we slip out of this rhythm, and don't get adequate quality sleep, our hormones get discombobulated; we cannot function properly, and our resilience is reduced.

QUICK NOTE

Sleep hygiene refers to cleaning up your sleep routine to make it more conducive to deep, satisfying rest. Here are a few things to consider:
- Avoid screen time (TV or computer) for at least one hour before bed.
- Disconnect Wi-Fi from your child's bedroom.
- Make the sleep environment dark. If you need a nightlight, ensure it's not too bright. Red and blue lights are best. Consider unplugging it once your child is asleep.
- Try magnesium and calcium before bed if your child has trouble settling.
- Try a calming tea, like catnip or lemon balm before bed.
- Establish a reliable, consistent bedtime routine.
- Be sure to connect with your children before they fall asleep. Talk to them about their day, or the breakfast you will have tomorrow, or what you hope to dream about. This can help them feel more secure as they slip off into slumber.

Section Summary

To improve resilience, the first order of business is to reduce social, environmental, and biological stress. This is step one of our two-step process. Short-term stress is something we can manage. It may even be supportive of our resilience. However, in this section I have addressed how constant underlying stress from any of these three sources puts undue pressure on our body and represents a barrier to resilience that needs managing if we desire good long-term health.

Most of Part One has been devoted to outlining the top biological stressors that I see in children, as well as offering some guidance for relieving them. These are not the only ones, but they are quite common and often overlooked. As I've emphasized, they have profound downstream effects on health and resilience, so making some shifts in your diet and lifestyle to relieve them can yield a massive health transformation.

Exploring the possible social, environmental, and biological stressors your child is exposed to, using a combination of keen observation, some lifestyle shifting, and possibly testing of blood, hair, saliva, stool, and urine with the help of your doctor, can help you determine what, if anything, might be interfering with optimal resilience for your child. Simply becoming aware of these common stressors and the symptoms they produce helps you support your child's health. Use this awareness to make changes, ask questions, and seek answers if you notice symptoms in your children.

Next we're going to turn to Part Two of the equation: giving the body what it needs to thrive, by learning and implementing the three core dietary strategies for building resilience.

PART TWO

THREE CORE DIETARY STRATEGIES FOR RAISING RESILIENCE

Introduction to Core Dietary Strategies

Once we have reduced stressors as described in Part One, Step Two for raising resilience includes implementing three core strategies which research shows support the body in its growth, development, and function.

Slowly adapting your feeding strategies to incorporate these concepts will help you simplify how you think about feeding your family and give you tangible ways to support their resilience. This section details each of the three strategies, giving thirty-six practical ways to make them come alive in your kitchen. You will find supportive lists in the appendices and sample recipes at the end of the book so you can get started right away.

The three core strategies are:
1. Maximize nutrient density
2. Control blood sugar
3. Support digestion

I've selected these as core strategies because new emerging medical research shows us that they lie upstream of so many processes, and because you can have a tremendous effect on them by altering how you do things in your kitchen. Optimizing these three things as best you can, and as often as you can, will give you the biggest bang for your buck because the trickle-down effect on health is so profound.

Raising Resilience

At the beginning of each core strategy you will find a Section Overview outlining the main message; following that, the details of why the strategy is so important. If you're feeling a little overwhelmed, go right to the list of practical action steps which you'll find at the end of each section along with a helpful summary. And for some helpful insights on how best to implement all the advice in *Raising Resilience*, you can refer to Part Four.

Core Strategy #1: Maximize Nutrient Density

Section Overview

Nutrients—amino acids, fatty acids, glucose, fibre, vitamins, minerals, phytochemicals, bacteria, and enzymes—essentially give us life. They feed our cells, activate chemical processes, eliminate waste, and bring important messages into our bodies.

Nutrients are different than calories. A calorie is a unit of energy associated with a food. A diet that is high in calories, yet low in nutrients, contributes to many mental illnesses, cardiovascular disease, diabetes, and obesity because, while calories give us energy, nutrients are the structural building blocks of our body and drivers of its function.

We improve nutrient density by choosing foods that are high in nutritional value, and avoiding foods that interfere with nutrient assimilation and action. In this way we make sure our bodies have all the nutrient requirements needed for optimal structure and function.

The Power of Nutrients

We have known for decades that certain nutrient deficiencies can lead to particular symptoms. Pellagra, for example, is a condition characterized by skin lesions, aggression, confusion, diarrhea, and dementia, all caused by a deficiency in vitamin B3. Most women who menstruate have felt the fatigue and moodiness brought on by low iron.

PART TWO: Three Core Dietary Strategies for Raising Resilience

Drawing on the understanding that nutrient deficiencies can cause real symptoms, integrative medical doctors, clinical nutritionists, naturopathic doctors, and orthomolecular doctors are noticing disease patterns, and are treating health conditions by improving nutrition. Autistic children, for example, are sometimes helped by adding supplements of critical brain vitamins and minerals.[49] Children with ADHD are often (not always) helped by increasing essential fatty acids.[50] People with anxiety are often helped with zinc, B6, and some omega 6 fatty acids.

Nutrients influence how we feel, function, behave, and develop. So the more nutrients we can bring in, the better.

You're likely aware that we need calcium for strong bones and teeth, and vitamin A for good eyesight. But let me give you a few examples to illustrate how the function of nutrients goes much deeper than that.

Various processes in the body, including energy production and tissue repair, produce molecules called free radicals. They are also produced when we are exposed to chemicals, foods, and stress. If we have too many free radicals floating around in our body they can diminish enzyme function, damage cells, increase inflammation, and damage DNA.[51] The damage they cause has been shown to contribute to a number of illnesses and conditions including cardiovascular disease, cancer, depression,[52] allergy, and ADHD.[53]

Luckily, nutrients including vitamins C, E, and A, the minerals zinc and selenium, CoQ10, and a host of chemicals found in plants like carotenoids, scavenge for free radicals, neutralizing them before they can cause damage. These nutrients are known as antioxidants. Our body also makes its own powerhouse antioxidants like glutathione and melatonin, but can only do so if nutrients like B12, folate, and the amino acid tryptophan are available. So you can see how, in their function as antioxidants, nutrients are key for disease prevention and proper function and growth.

Raising Resilience

Here's another example. Methylation is a complex process in the body by which a compound called a methyl group is donated to another molecule. You can think of methylation as an on-off switch; many processes and compounds in the body need to be methylated in order to either start working or stop working. Here are some examples:
- Certain genes need to be methylated to be turned on or off.
- Certain hormones and neurotransmitters need to be methylated.
- Metals such as mercury need to be methylated before they can be flushed from the body.
- Inflammation is partially controlled by methylation.
- Histamine production is turned off by methylation.
- Glutathione, one of our master antioxidants, is created and then recycled through the process of methylation.

Many steps are involved in methylation, but nutrients play a significant role. Without enough nutrients like B12, methionine, B6, magnesium, glycine, and zinc, the methylation process can slow down considerably. On the flip side, insufficient omega 3 fatty acids, choline, zinc, and vitamin C can contribute to over-methylation.

The recent discovery of methylation as an on-off switch is slowly revolutionizing how doctors can treat dozens of chronic ailments using nutrition to regulate the methylation process. It's a delicate dance that requires proper testing but for parents it illustrates and emphasizes the importance of nutrients.

These are just two examples to make the point that the underlying biochemistry which keeps us healthy requires a steady supply of nutrients. Here are a few more examples:
- Thyroid hormones require iodine and selenium to be created and function properly.
- Neurotransmitters and enzymes are built out of amino acids (protein).

PART TWO: Three Core Dietary Strategies for Raising Resilience

- Stomach acid production requires adequate zinc and vitamin C.

There are plenty more examples but the point has been made: nutrients build structure and drive function; nutrient deficiencies lead to system breakdown.

Nutrients also have another important role to play in our health: they clean house. Nutrients sweep our bodies clean of no-longer-needed hormones, chemicals, and cholesterol and, as you just learned, neutralize free radicals before they can destabilize healthy cells. From a "cleaning" standpoint, nutrient density has never been so important. A 2005 study in the United States found 287 chemicals in umbilical cord blood, including known carcinogens, nervous system toxins, and hormone mimickers.[54] The 2013 Canadian report published by Environmental Defence put the number at 137 different carcinogens, metals, and nervous system toxicants.[55] Children today are typically born with a high toxic load, and then exposed to an ever increasing number of destabilizing elements, which leaves them with a greater need for nutrients.

Proper function, stable moods, quality sleep, strong bones, ability to focus and learn, and more, all starts with optimizing our nutrient intake. Because children are in such a rapid state of growth, with cells multiplying and systems developing, they require a great deal of nutrients every single day. Start to implement my guidelines to improve their nutrient density. If you continue to see troubling symptoms, there are several appendices at the back of the book to help you do some detective work to match symptoms and behaviours with common nutritional deficiencies. Use this information to better understand your child's body, begin tailoring a custom diet, and confidently initiate a conversation with your healthcare team about targeted testing and supplementation. See Appendix F, H, and K.

For many families though, simply increasing the nutrient density of the diet using the following strategies will be enough to yield massive improvement in resilience. As cells are better nourished and chemical processes are revved up, the body can function better.

Nutrient Density

Embracing the concept of nutrient density will help you become efficient with your time and dollars, while being sure to get all the important nutrients covered. This section outlines how to do that.

Examples of nutrient-poor foods versus their more nutrient-dense alternatives:

Less Nutrient-Dense	More Nutrient-Dense
White flour	Nut flour, bean flour, coconut flour, whole grain flour
White sugar	Molasses, honey, Sucanat
Hot dog	Pure grass-fed meat sausage with no additives or fillers
Freezie, popsicle	Homemade fruit popsicles
Ranch dip	Vegetable sticks, homemade seed cookies with hummus dip or sour cream
Low fat flavoured yogurt	Full fat plain yogurt or kefir with berries
Canned fruit in syrup	A piece of fruit
Breakfast cereal	Cooked oatmeal (not instant) with hemp and chia seeds, topped with berries
Bouillon	Homemade chicken stock
Soda pop	Fermented water, kefir soda
Flavoured sweetened yogurt for kids	Plain whole yogurt with fruit and honey

Here's an example: Two breakfasts that might look the same but, due to minor changes, rate very differently on a nutrient density scale.

Breakfast #1: Two factory farmed eggs fried in margarine, grocery store bacon, a blueberry muffin with margarine, and a commercial brand of peanut butter.

VERSUS

PART TWO: Three Core Dietary Strategies for Raising Resilience

Breakfast #2: Two farm fresh eggs from pastured hens, fried in coconut oil, grass-fed and additive-free bacon or homemade sausage, gluten-free quinoa blueberry muffin topped with all natural almond butter.

What's the difference? Nutrient density. These two meals might look similar, but they're totally different in terms of nutritional value.

Breakfast #2 is higher in healthy fatty acids, lower in chemicals, additives, and destructive fats, less irritating to the digestive and immune systems, and higher in nutrients. It will be more a little more expensive, but it's actually the best way to stretch a dollar because it will fill the tank longer due to its fibre, increased nutrients, and healthy fat content.

Nutrient Categories

Some authors and health agencies warn us against thinking about foods as nutrients. The approach has been called "nutritionism," and the caution is that this approach distances us from the food we eat. I agree that we should keep our eye on the big picture, connect with our food, and teach our kids to do the same. However, I also think, as parents who are in charge of choosing what our kids eat, a nutrient-focused approach can be quite helpful. While I don't talk about nutrients with my young children, I do instruct parents to think about them as they relate to body function, so that they can make sure everything is being covered.

Allow me to go a little "nutritionalistic" on you, and introduce you to the eight nutrient groups you need to have on your radar. Then we'll talk about the foods you find them in, and how to combine them in healthful and delicious ways. You can also refer to Appendix A and B for food and nutrient lists.

First, in a way, I'd like you to throw The Food Pyramid, your My Plate, and your Canada's Food Guide out the window. They do not give you a complete enough picture of what current research shows us a body needs to be resilient.

Instead, I want you to become familiar with eight main nutrient categories, that is, eight categories of nutrients that need to be covered every day in order to call your diet nutrient-dense. Focusing on these groups will make sure your kids become well nourished, not only well fed.

These eight categories can be split into two groups: macronutrients and micronutrients.

Macronutrients are the fats, proteins, and carbohydrates. They provide calories. The micronutrients (vitamins, minerals, phytochemicals, enzymes, and bacteria), create the magic in our bodies; they're the catalysts that make everything happen. They are regulators. They are drivers and without them, all processes in the body grind to a halt. Micronutrient deficiency can lead to sluggish metabolism, poor detoxification, poor digestion, weak immune function, weak bone structure, and a general lack of resilience.

While macronutrients are easy to access and easy to recognize, the micronutrients are dependent on the health of the soil in which the food was grown and, many are easily destroyed by heat, processing, and time. We all know the reality of our modern food supply. The mono-cropping, shipping, storage, extraction, processing, and chemicals involved lead to a modern diet that is sorely lacking in these essential micronutrients. We have to increase our efforts to make sure they get covered.

A nutrient-dense diet is one that includes all of these categories on a regular basis. Bringing these nutrient groups to the forefront of your attention, and finding creative ways to get them into your children will help you raise resilience. Look in the appendix for charts detailing which foods will supply these nutrients, and to the sample recipes section for creative ideas on how to cook with them.

PART TWO: Three Core Dietary Strategies for Raising Resilience

Before getting into the strategies for integrating this core strategy into your life, I want now to clear up some of the confusion that surrounds these nutrient categories.

Healthy Fat

There are numerous misconceptions when it comes to fat, because our understanding of what fat does in the body is evolving. If you want the abbreviated notes on fats, including which ones to use, skip down to page 75. Continue reading here if you want more details.

Facts about Fat:
- Fat is a component of every single cell in your body.
- The brain is 60% fat.
- The heart muscle is nourished by fat.
- Fats are needed for proper absorption of fat-soluble vitamins (A, D, E, and K), which in turn are essential for proper growth, immune function, digestive health, and more.
- Fats are involved in hormone production which is essential to prevent things like acne, poor fertility and sex drive, PMS, depression, and mood swings.

Quality dietary fat is not causing the childhood obesity epidemic. Research is clearly showing that this has more to do with sugar, eating patterns, microbiota, poor quality processed fat, carbohydrates, and chemicals.[56] Good quality dietary fat is necessary for good health. Without enough, our brains, immune systems, nervous systems, hormones, bones, and teeth do not develop or function properly.

Dietary fat gets broken down into fatty acids through the process of digestion. There are two categories of fatty acids: unsaturated and saturated. Both provide essential value to the body and should together make up about 30% of your child's calories.

Let's start with the unsaturated category.

Raising Resilience

There are two families of unsaturated fatty acids: polyunsaturated, and monounsaturated. Vegetable and seed oils tend to be high in polyunsaturated fatty acids, while olive oil, avocado, and certain nuts tend to be high in monounsaturated fatty acids.

Monounsaturated fatty acids have been shown to have a very positive effect on health, such as reducing risk of cancer and heart disease. Including cold pressed olive oil, nuts, and avocados in the diet is the best way to get enough of this type of fat.

Within the polyunsaturated subgroup we find a non-essential group and an essential group. Non-essential fatty acids are polyunsaturated fatty acids that the body can make as long as all the factors are in place to do so. Essential fatty acids (EFAs) are those the body has to get through food or supplements.

Omega 3 and omega 6 are types of essential polyunsaturated fatty acids. Both are important, particularly during childhood, when cells are replicating so rapidly.

About 60% of the brain is fat and 94% of the brain's fat is made up of an omega 3 essential fatty acid called DHA or Docosahexaenoic acid. EFAs are also important for immune health, cardiovascular function, eye development, and skin health, and they help regulate inflammation. A child needs a steady supply of EFAs to develop optimally. And remember, the body can't make these fatty acids; we have to get them from food. Many prenatal vitamins and infant formulas are now including them. They remain just as important later in childhood.

It's important to understand the influence of essential fatty acids on inflammation. Omega 6 fatty acids begin a cascade of processes that result in inflammation. Omega 3 fatty acids do the opposite; they initiate anti-inflammatory pathways. Keeping the proper ratio between the two is important. Too much 6, not enough 3, or an insufficiency of both has been implicated in just about every chronic disease including:

PART TWO: Three Core Dietary Strategies for Raising Resilience

- allergies
- fatigue
- hyperactivity
- dyslexia
- weight gain
- eczema
- poor immune function
- mood swings
- asthma
- depression
- cancer
- skin disorders
- behaviour disorders
- ADD/ADHD
- arthritis
- memory problems
- heart disease
- diabetes

Experts disagree about what the optimal ratio of 6 to 3 is, although it is likely somewhere between 1:1 and 4:1 (that's omega 6:omega 3). Current estimates are that the average American gets about 20:1.[57]

Shortly, you'll learn how to ensure proper intake of EFAs for the best absorption and benefit, but first let's turn to the second category of important fats, saturated fat.

Saturated fatty acids stay solid at room temperature. They are found mostly in animal foods, but are also in tropical oils like coconut and palm.

Saturated fat, and the cholesterol that often accompanies it, are also critical for children. Note, there is no cholesterol in coconut oil or palm oil. Cholesterol is only found in animal foods. The body does use saturated fat to make cholesterol, which is why the two are often talked about together.

Saturated fatty acids:
- provide stiffness and integrity to cell membranes
- help the body absorb calcium into bones
- protect the liver and kidneys
- enhance the immune system
- help the body properly utilize EFAs
- nourish the heart muscle
- help digestion
- provide energy

While unsaturated fats such as vegetable oils break down in heat, saturated fats can withstand heat without losing their healthy properties. Because of that, fats that are highly saturated such as butter, virgin coconut oil, red palm oil, and organic lard are good choices for high heat cooking.

Important to know: Toxins accumulate in animal fat. So, if you're buying fat that comes from an animal, choose the organic version whenever possible.

To be sure you get all the different types of fatty acids represented in your child's diet, see page 60 for a list of the best oils to use in your cooking.

Protein
Protein is involved in just about every function of the body. Children need a consistent supply to build the body's structure (muscles, connective tissue, etc.), create enzymes and hormones, build the immune system, and complete thousands of other jobs.

Along with the fatty acids you just learned about, proteins also provide an important component of cell walls. Cells are the basic unit of the body; they work together to create tissues, which work

PART TWO: Three Core Dietary Strategies for Raising Resilience

together to create organs, which work together to create systems. So without adequate protein, body systems cannot function properly because cells will not be healthy.

Proteins are long strings of amino acids that get broken down through the process of digestion into single amino acids. Think of a tower of Lego. Each piece is an amino acid. The tower of Lego is a protein.

Varying combinations of amino acids create different types of protein. Gluten, for example, is a type of protein consisting of a specific configuration of amino acids.

Non-essential amino acids are those the body can make if sufficient raw material is present. Essential amino acids (there are nine of them) are those the body cannot make; we have to get them from food.

Sources of complete protein:
- red meat
- eggs
- organ meat
- tofu
- miso
- nut butters with whole grain
- whole milk (cow, sheep, or goat)
- all dairy cheeses
- chia
- fish
- chicken
- legumes and grains together
- tempeh
- hemp seeds
- yogurt
- goat cheese
- edamame
- quinoa

Whether plant or animal protein is the better choice, along with how much protein is needed for optimal health, are issues fraught with controversy. Based on my research and clinical experience, I have found that a varied diet which includes quality plant and animal protein offers a child the best diversity of nutrients. Again, the key is to understand your body and test foods out against your own particular physiology, and that of your children. Some people seem to fare better with more meat, others with more plants. What everyone seems to agree on, though, is that quality is important.

I find that most children do well with about 30% of their diet made up of good quality protein.

Carbohydrates

This macronutrient, abundant in starchy vegetables, grains, dairy, and legumes is a source of energy for cells. When a carbohydrate enters the digestive tract, it gets broken down into glucose, which then enters the bloodstream and gets shuttled into cells by the hormone and insulin, along with the help of chromium. There, in the cells, the glucose gets turned into energy.

Fibre is a type of carbohydrate that is not broken down by the digestive process. Instead, fibre helps "sweep" the body of waste and it feeds beneficial bacteria in the colon.

I recommend, for the average child, that about 40% of their diet be quality carbohydrates, which includes about 20 to 30 gram of fibre a day. Choosing appropriate carbohydrates will be discussed more in depth when we talk about blood sugar.

Vitamins

Vitamins do not bring calories into the body but they are essential for all sorts of processes including immune function, proper digestion and absorption, and healthy bone structure. Some vitamins are fat-soluble, meaning they need to be absorbed into fat before the body can use them. They can also be stored in fat for later use. Fat soluble vitamins include vitamins A, D, E, and K. Some vitamins, like vitamins C and all the Bs, are water soluble—they are absorbed right into the blood but cannot be stored. The body also makes a few vitamins—we can convert sunlight into vitamin D and our gut bacteria make small amounts of vitamin K.

Minerals

Minerals have a similar function to vitamins, the main difference being that minerals are inorganic substances that come from soil and water; they cannot be made by the body and the amount in foods is dependent on the soil and water with which the foods were grown. Sadly, many foods have become deficient in vital minerals which makes what we read on food labels and in nutrition charts largely theoretical.

Phytonutrients (also known as Phytochemicals)

"Phyto" means plant. Phytonutrients are nutrients found in plants. There are hundreds of them, with very long names, and we are still discovering how they affect the body.

Many of the phytonutrients fall into the category of antioxidant, the free radical chasing nutrients we talked about earlier. You'll recall that chemicals, pollution, and stress, as well as natural processes like metabolism, create free radicals in the body that can do damage to other cells if they are not neutralized by antioxidants.

While food from animals supply a few antioxidants as well as some of the building blocks needed for the body to create its own such as zinc,[58] B vitamins,[59] and vitamin D,[60] plants provide us with a significantly higher direct source of antioxidants.[61] This is partly what makes plants an important part of any healthy diet.

Phytochemicals provide a whole host of other health benefits ranging from improving heart health and immune function to preventing cancer and cognitive decline. It can be helpful to think of phytochemical function in terms of their colour. When you "eat the rainbow," you ensure you are getting some of every family of phytonutrients represented in your diet.

- Red – Lycopene: This is found in red foods like red peppers, guava, papaya, watermelon, pink grapefruit, mangos, tomatoes, and watermelon. It is a type of carotenoid that is heart protective, helps with male fertility, and prevents aging of the skin. It also helps prevent diabetes and osteoporosis.
- Orange/Yellow – Cartenoids: You will find carotenoids in foods like sweet potatoes, yellow peppers, yellow squash, carrots, and melons. Lutein, beta-carotene, and zeaxanthin are just a few of the carotenoids. They are helpful with eyesight, and may assist in preventing cancer.
- Green – Chlorophyll: Chlorophyll is the green pigment found in plants. It cleanses and builds the blood, and helps detoxify the body. It aids in promoting good bacteria and is a major antioxidant. It supports the immune system and fights infection, and may help protect against cancer. Good sources of chlorophyll are green leafy vegetables such as kale, spinach, broccoli, parsley, cilantro, and wheat grass.
- Blue/Purple/Black – Anthocyanins: Anthocyanins are major antioxidants that help protect the blood, brain, and nervous system, and support the growth of collagen and connective tissue. They benefit our eyesight, and have heart protective and cancer preventative properties. Blueberries, red and purple grapes, raspberries, black currants, blackberries, black raspberries, pomegranate, red cabbage, and eggplant are all good sources. So is red wine. The richest sources of anthocyanins are found in black foods like black beans, black sesame, blackberries, black rice, and black cherry tomatoes.

PART TWO: Three Core Dietary Strategies for Raising Resilience

Catechins are another important phytochemical. They are found in green and black tea, and chocolate. All catechins are potent antioxidants. They are heart protective, improve cognitive function, and protect against cancer.

The current recommendation for our children is that they get 7 to 13 servings per day of colourful fresh fruits and vegetables to supply the 25,000 types of phytonutrients needed for good health. This can be a challenge! Check out the ideas in the Recipes for Resilience section as well as the supplemental recommendations on my website (www.jesssherman.com) to help you along.

Enzymes

Enzymes are proteins that function as catalysts in the body; they initiate and speed up all chemical processes. Without enzymes, hundreds of chemical reactions cannot be completed, and if this happens, functions grind to a halt.

We require a steady supply of over 3,000 different enzymes for optimal health. There are two types: digestive enzymes and metabolic enzymes.

Metabolic enzymes function inside cells. They speed up metabolic reactions and are responsible for cellular growth, energy production, and even DNA production and expression.

Digestive enzymes function in the digestive tract to support digestive processes. They work in a lock-and-key fashion with various substrates. The enzyme, lipase, acts upon fats (lipids); pepsin acts on protein; amylase acts on carbohydrate; lactase acts on lactose.

The pancreas releases enzymes when we eat but the enzymes in food are largely destroyed by heat and degrade with time. So ample fresh raw fruits and vegetables and living foods like sprouts and fermented foods are our best direct sources.

Bacteria

Somewhere in the range of 100 trillion microbes (bacteria) from at least 1,000 different species inhabit our bodies.[62] They are emerging as substantial partners in just about every bodily function.[63] They are involved in immune function, metabolism, digestion, detoxification, cognitive function, DNA expression ... among other things.[64] The relatively new discovery of our symbiotic relationship with microbes is revolutionizing how we view the body, health, disease, and resilience. We will talk much more about bacteria when we review the third core strategy, supporting digestion, starting on page 108.

We inherit bacteria from our mothers through the birth process and we acquire more in the early stages of life. Raw and living foods like those mentioned with regards to enzymes are our best dietary sources of bacteria.

The nutrients needed for detoxification, growth, body structure, and function are found abundantly in quality, whole foods. But, of course, having a nutrient-dense diet requires that we overcome some very real obstacles. Access to nutrient-rich food grown and raised on good quality soil is diminishing as the quality of our soils is depleting, access to poor quality food is increasing; and stressful and busy family schedules often exclude time for high quality home cooked meals, not to mention that kids often are picky.

While getting calories into our kids might be fairly straight forward, including an ample supply of healthy nutrients can be a difficult task. And, as you've learned, it is the nutrients more so than the calories that drive growth and development. It's one thing to understand what your perfect diet should be, it's entirely another to figure out how to access quality food and get that great stuff into your kids. So let's talk strategies and solutions.

PART TWO: Three Core Dietary Strategies for Raising Resilience

Fifteen Ways to Maximize Nutrient Density

1. Incorporate Healthy Fats into Your Cooking

   To make sure you get sufficient amounts of all the important fatty acids, use a variety of the following healthy fats, alternating amongst them for diversity.

   For high-heat cooking like sautéing and frying, highly saturated and monounsaturated fats should be your preferred choice. The following are suitable for heating. The first three will bring mostly saturated fat into the diet. Lard, duck fat, and red palm oil are nice mixtures of saturated and mono-unsaturated. The rest are high in unsaturated fat:
   - butter
   - ghee (butter oil that has had the protein taken out)
   - coconut oil
   - duck fat
   - lard from grass-fed pigs (you'll likely have to get this straight from a local small farm, if you have one in your area, not from the grocery store.)
   - red palm oil
   - sesame oil
   - avocado oil
   - rice bran oil
   - cold-pressed olive oil

For baking, use butter, coconut oil, ghee, red palm oil, moderate amounts of rice bran oil, avocado oil, and sunflower oil.

For dressings and toppings, use flax oil and walnut oil; these fats should not be heated. Also, keep in mind that while cold-pressed olive oil, sesame oil, and sunflower oil may be heated, their health benefits are best preserved if they too are used raw.

As a supplement, use purified fish oil, cod liver oil, and butter oil when needed (see Appendix F for guidance on picking supplements).

I also suggest that you reduce your intake of vegetable and seed oils such as corn, canola, cottonseed, and soy oils as they are counterproductive to raising resilience. You might find this surprising, but I suggest you reduce these oils for four reasons:

- They are normally extracted from plants using high pressure and heat, which can alter their chemistry. If ever choosing vegetable or seed oils, be absolutely sure they are cold-pressed.
- The chemical, hexane, is often used in the extraction process, the residue of which has been found in the oil. While levels found in oils are quite low, they can add up and the health effects are still largely unknown.
- The crops used to make the bulk of vegetable oils (corn, soy, cotton) are often genetically modified, unless labelled organic. We have yet to fully understand the long term health consequences of the genetic modification process but, as mentioned in Part One, there is significant evidence that raises cause for concern.
- Vegetable and seed oils are a source of omega 6 fatty acids, the kind we tend to get too much of in our diets and which stimulates the process of inflammation. It's better to use other cooking oils and get your omega 6s from foods that provide a more balanced ratio of omega 3:6 like those listed in the appendix. Even the healthy seed oils mentioned above, like rice bran and sesame, should be used in moderation as they are high in omega 6 fatty acids. They are included as healthy fats because they also contain significant monounsaturated fatty acids.

QUICK NOTES ABOUT FAT

Coconut oil is a particularly helpful fat as it contains lauric acid, a fatty acid which nourishes the immune system and has antimicrobial and anti-parasitic qualities that help keep digestion flowing smoothly. Coconut milk also provides these benefits.

As well, experiment with red palm oil. Coming in at about fifty percent saturated and fifty percent unsaturated (which is similar to good quality lard), it has been shown to reduce oxidative stress, cholesterol, the risk of atherosclerosis, blood pressure, and improve immune function, possible due to its high concentration of beta carotene, vitamin E, and unsaturated fat.[65]

2. Avoid All Trans Fats

Trans fat is a type of fat created when hydrogen has been added to an unsaturated fat to make it act like a saturated fat (i.e. solid and shelf stable). While some trans fats occur naturally in food and are managed by our bodies, manufactured trans fat is so dangerous it's astounding (and sad) that it's still in our food supply.

Trans fat has been associated with a whole host of problems including:
- cancer
- atherosclerosis
- diabetes
- obesity
- immune system dysfunction
- low birth-weight babies
- birth defects
- decreased visual acuity
- sterility
- difficulty in lactation
- problems with bones and tendons
- sexual dysfunction
- increased blood cholesterol
- immune system disorders

Raising Resilience

Trans fat is counterproductive to raising resilience because it literally takes the place of healthier fats in cellular structure. Think of your child's cell walls like a parking lot; if unhealthy trans fatty acids take up all the parking spaces, there's no room left for the healthy fatty acids. If this happens during a period of growth, such as childhood, it can lead to poor cellular development.

At this point in Canada, it is perfectly legal to label something as trans fat free if it has less than 0.5 g. trans fat per serving. That means, 2 tablespoons of peanut butter labelled trans fat free might have as much as 3 g. of trans fat. This from a product you thought was trans fat-free. Yes, apparently, it is perfectly legal. Check the ingredients list on that peanut butter to find out if there are trans fats in the product. If it contains hydrogenated or partially hydrogenated vegetable oils, it contains trans fat. Don't rely on the marketing and health claims on the packaging.

How much trans fat is too much, you ask? Health Canada takes a peculiar stance; they recommend that trans fat intake be no more than one percent of your total fat intake. I find it strange to think of your trans fat intake as a ratio of your total fat intake, as the two have nothing to do with each other from a health standpoint. Also, growing children need more fat in their diets. So this would mean the acceptable level of trans fat for children would be higher than that of an adult. This is also misleading, since trans fats are particularly harmful for children since they are in a rapid state of growth.

To reiterate, keep trans fats out of the diet by avoiding hydrogenated oil, partially hydrogenated oil, modified fats, and esterified oils (non-hydrogenated margarines).

3. Learn to Ferment Your Own Foods
   You might be thinking that this sounds like a stretch, wondering, "Will my kids eat that? It'll take too much time! It's too scary and complicated."

PART TWO: Three Core Dietary Strategies for Raising Resilience

Rest assured, it takes very little time, can be super tasty and kid friendly, there are only a few things to know, and it is the best way to get those enzymes and probiotic bacteria in. Fermented foods are truly super foods and learning to ferment is well worth the effort. We'll talk more about it in the section on digestion. In the meantime, you can often find fermented foods like kombucha, lacto-fermented sauerkraut and pickles and kefir in smaller grocery stores or markets. Look for them in the refrigerated section and watch for additives—truly fermented foods do not contain gelatin, pectin, gums, or vinegar. You can also find great recipes and quick tips on how to start fermenting your own foods in the sample recipes section and on my website.

4. Try Cooking with Seaweed
   Seaweed contains a wealth of highly bio-available amino acids, vitamins, and minerals including calcium, iron, iodine, and B vitamins. Here are a few ways to use seaweed:
   - When cooking any grain or soup, add a one-inch piece of kombu or wakame seaweed to the water. The nutrients from the sea vegetable will seep into the food, creating a more nutritious meal without altering the flavour.
   - When cooking beans, place some kombu in the water. This helps break down the fiber in the beans making them easier to digest and less likely to produce gas.
   - Mix kelp powder or flakes into your salt dish to sprinkle freely on foods. Kelp has a salty flavour that blends nicely with rock or sea salt while adding valuable minerals.
   - Try arame seaweed, which has a noodle-like texture and can be nicely mixed with rice-noodles in an Asian-type salad.

5. Super-Enrich Your Grains

    Instead of using water to cook your grains, use homemade broth or a mixture of water and broth. Homemade bone broth is full of minerals and nutrients soothing to the intestinal lining and helpful for digestion. The goodness from the broth will be absorbed into the grain as it cooks, giving the grains, and your meal, a flavour and nutrient boost. You'll find several broth recipes at the back in the Recipes for Resilience section. You can also try adding some coconut cream to you cooking water for added healthy fat.

6. Try Nutritive Teas

    Nettle, turmeric, Pau D'Arco, catnip, peppermint, and rosehip are some of my favourites. They are mild tasting and can be used as is, or as a base for another beverage (like a smoothie or hot chocolate). You can even swap out water for some of the milder teas in recipes like pancake batter, or add them to soups. Taste the tea and use your culinary judgement as sometimes teas will alter taste and color. Peppermint tea works well with hot chocolate, nettle (which is high in iron) works well in soups, and Pau D'Arco is great in or with almost anything as it has a very mild taste. Rosehip is nice mixed with fruit juice and frozen into a popsicle. Also, experiment with keeping a mason jar of brewed nutritive tea in the fridge, as a refreshing alternative to juice or water.

7. Use Hemp Seeds

    Hemp seeds are high in protein, iron, and fatty acids. Unlike most other seeds, hemp seeds are low in phytic acid, a nutrient that can bind to minerals like zinc and iron and pull them out of the body. Avoid going overboard, though, as they do contain quite a bit of the inflammatory omega 6 fatty acids. Balance

PART TWO: Three Core Dietary Strategies for Raising Resilience

them out by ensuring you are getting omega 3s, as indicated in Appendix F. Toss hemp seeds into salads, sprinkle them on top of cereal, bake them into muffins and bread, or grind them into smoothies. Hemp seeds, also called hemp hearts, can be eaten whole or ground. Store them in the fridge to preserve their fragile fatty acids.

8. Join a Community Supported Agriculture (CSA) Group and Visit Local Farmers' Markets

    In an ideal world we'd all have ample year-round access to affordable, fresh, colourful, local organic vegetables grown in lush soils, and pastured meat and eggs from farms conscientious about how their animals eat and live. This food is the most nutrient-dense as the nutrition has not been eroded by the burden of storage and travel. While that is not always possible, the best way to access this type of highly nutrient-dense food is to buy local as much as possible.

    CSA is a business model that connects farmers directly to consumers. A quick internet search will likely find one servicing your area. The model usually involves prepaying a local farmer for a season's worth of produce. Prices are generally reasonable. Some farms even support work-shares (i.e. you volunteer time on the farm in exchange for produce).

    Joining a Community Supported Agriculture group is a fantastic way to:
    - support your local food economy and keep passionate farmers in business
    - access maximum nutrition and enzyme levels by getting the freshest possible produce
    - learn about new foods you might be unfamiliar with, including heritage varieties that are loaded with phytochemicals and flavours
    - get great quality, affordable food

If you don't want to, or can't pay for a CSA, check out your local farmers' market and talk to the vendors there. Most will sell to you directly from the farm gate at reasonable prices; some will even be open to trades and home delivery.

9. Join a Food Co-op (Buying Club)
Food Co-op buying clubs are another great way to save money while getting good quality. You don't have to be a store to buy in bulk and get wholesale prices. Buying from a co-op allows you to buy straight from the distributor, cutting the store (and its mark-up) out of the loop. They are a great place to buy things like dried fruit, nuts, flour, seeds, grains, and baking ingredients. Some co-ops offer more diversity and better prices than others, so shop around.

Most co-ops do have a minimum required purchase, but if you get a couple of friends together and place an order every few months you can easily meet the minimum. For a distributor in your area, simply do an internet search and contact them for details. You'll save a bundle and have food delivered right to your door.

10. Reduce Sugar and Swap Out Your Sweeteners
We've already touched on sugar and will talk much more about it when dive into Core Strategy #2. But understand that refined sugar strips the body of nutrients and contains little itself. Later on, you'll learn about low glycemic sweeteners to try, but you can also experiment with molasses, palm sugar, Sucanat, rapadura, and coconut nectar. They cause a little less damage and contain some minerals.

11. Swap the Salt
Table salt is almost completely sodium chloride, excessive levels of which can be damaging to our health. Switch to Himalayan

PART TWO: Three Core Dietary Strategies for Raising Resilience

rock salt or unrefined sea salt to get a broader spectrum of essential minerals while curbing your intake of sodium chloride. You can even enhance the mineral content of your salt further by mixing it with kelp flakes, which also have a salty taste (see Recipes for Resilience section).

12. Boost Veggie Intake
    I know, boosting the veggies can be tricky for some parents. Here are some ideas:
    - Grind up veggies into sauces, stews, and muffins. Carrots, zucchini, spinach, chard, squash, sweet potato, and pumpkin are the easiest to add in.
    - Use pumpkin and squash as a binder in muffins or thickener in sauces.
    - Incorporate a dried veggie powder into smoothies and popsicles.
    - Make a habit of putting chopped raw veggies on the table at dinner (or have them available right before dinner when the kids come wandering into the kitchen). After school is also a great time for raw veggie snacks. Carrots, cucumbers, sugar snap peas, and celery are the easiest to have on hand. Also try peeled kohlrabi, jicama, and daikon radish if you're feeling adventurous.

13. Swap Out the Flours
    When baking, try replacing wheat with some of the nutrient-dense gluten-free flours like teff, buckwheat, sorghum, amaranth, and almond. These flours behave quite differently than wheat flour, so be ready to experiment. You'll find more tips on using gluten-free flours in Appendix H.

14. Invest in Good Kitchen Equipment
    Get a crock pot (slow cooker), and learn how to use it. This is

one piece of kitchen equipment that has made my life so much easier, and I promise it will do the same for you. All you do is load it and leave it. What could be better?

From a nutritional standpoint, when cooking meat, a long, slow cook will preserve the healthy fats. If you've spent the money to buy quality grass-fed meat, cooking it in a slow cooker will preserve the health and flavour of the food you've spent your hard-earned dollars on.

Also invest in a high-powered blender if you haven't already. A blender that has a motor powerful enough to really pulverize food so it gets smooth allows you to jam-pack your smoothies, soups, and even batters with all kinds of healthy goodies.

15. Incorporate Targeted Quality Supplements

You're certainly not alone if you find it an overwhelming task at times to get enough quality nutrients into your child. Quality supplements can relieve some of the pressure, and help ensure you're getting the bases covered.

Furthermore, as touched on briefly already, some kids might be showing symptoms indicating that they need extra nutrition, beyond what is realistic to get through food alone. Refer to appendices F and K to discern how certain deficiencies could relate to particular symptoms you might be dealing with.

When it comes to supplementation, it's always best to work with a practitioner who can evaluate and understand your child's particular needs. But if you want to experiment on your own, be very careful to choose only top quality. You need your supplements to be highly absorbable, come from quality raw materials, and be purified of toxins. Otherwise they are not worth spending money on. See Appendix I for some advice on picking supplements.

PART TWO: Three Core Dietary Strategies for Raising Resilience

Section Summary

Nutrients are critical building blocks for the structure and function of our bodies. They're also critical players in our ability to detoxify and clear our bodies of waste. If you are not seeing behaviour, digestive, sleep, skin, immune, or respiratory symptoms, then all you need to do is stick to a nutrient-dense diet and get the main eight nutrient categories into your child as much as possible. The fifteen ways mentioned in this section will help you with that.

If, on the other hand, you are seeing some troubling symptoms, and you want to try to figure out how food might be contributing, you'll need to do a little work tailoring your nutrient-dense diet to your child's specific needs. You might be dealing with underlying genetic conditions, food allergy, or nutrient deficiencies that need supplementation and collaboration with health care providers. See appendices E, F, and K at the end of the book to help guide your conversations with practitioners who understand the connection between symptoms and nutrition.

> *QUICK NOTE*
> Check food labels to avoid these top unclean ingredients:
> - non-organic or hydrogenated soy, corn, cottonseed, or canola oils
> - monosodium glutamate (MSG)
> - hydrolysed protein (which is MSG in another form)
> - calcium disodium EDTA
> - polysorbate 80
> - bisphenol-A (BPA), especially associated with fatty or acidic food like tomatoes and coconut milk (note that this one is not listed in the ingredients list—it is found in the lining of cans and in some plastics)
> - artificial sweeteners
> - tertiary butyl hydroquinone (TBHQ)
> - Butylated hydroxyanisole (BHA) and butylated hydroxytoluene (BHT)

- brominated vegetable oils (BVO), often found in sports drinks
- artificial numbered food dyes

QUICK NOTE
Is organic worth it?

Buying organic food as much as possible is worth the extra money if you can do it. Children are small and they are in a rapid state of cellular development. This means they are particularly at risk from the harmful effects of chemicals. When chemicals are tested and determined to be safe, they are not tested for these particular circumstances of childhood. They are also tested in isolation, whereas they are always consumed in combination. We do not yet fully know the extent of the stress this "cocktail effect" can have on a child's body. Chemicals and pesticides have been shown in some cases to trigger allergies, disrupt the endocrine system, and cause various other issues relating to mood, sleep, skin, bowels, and behaviour.[66] The Pesticide Action Network of North America (PANNA) has compiled a lot of research about the dangers of pesticides. They are a great resource for finding out more about what's on or in our food, and how to avoid it. Visit www.panna.org.

Eating clean food does not have to break the bank. If you can only afford a limited number of organic foods, refer to the Environmental Working Group's yearly tests. Each year they come out with their Clean Fifteen and Dirty Dozen lists; they include the foods (produce only) that contain the least amount of chemicals and those that contain the most. Access the latest version on the Environmental Working Group website at www.ewg.org. By following their guide you will cut your pesticide consumption by eighty percent.

PART TWO: Three Core Dietary Strategies for Raising Resilience

Core Strategy #2: Control Blood Sugar

Section Overview

You've already learned the basics of how excessive sugar reduces resilience because of its effect on blood sugar. But blood sugar also influences the health and function of the nervous system, immune system, hormones, bacteria, and inflammation. This section helps you understand how controlling blood sugar helps prevent and resolve health issues such as overweight and obesity, depression, anxiety, moodiness, hyperactivity, aggression, inability to fall or stay asleep, poor appetite, chronic infections, candida overgrowth, fatigue, inattention, and impulsivity. You'll learn how to identify symptoms of poor blood sugar control, and what steps to take to support resilience by keeping blood sugar stable.

The huge return that attending to blood sugar gives is why it is one of the first areas I work on with most of my clients, regardless of the particular symptoms they are dealing with. If you want to skip over the details, you can go right to the strategies which start on page 93.

Understanding Carbohydrates

To understand blood sugar we have to focus in on one of the three macronutrients you were introduced to earlier — carbohydrates. A carbohydrate is a made up of different types of sugar molecules (saccharides). The body uses these molecules to create energy.

Let's start at the beginning and follow a carbohydrate through the body. Carbohydrates enter the body from foods like grains, bread, muffins, dairy, fruits, legumes, and vegetables. Through the process of digestion, they get pulled apart into the three simplest forms of sugar: glucose, fructose, and galactose. These sugars are then transported through the digestive wall and into the bloodstream.

Glucose is a form of sugar that is ready to be used. All cells of the body are able to create energy from glucose. Galactose is eventually transformed into glucose for use, and we'll expand on fructose more when we talk about fruit. Let's first focus on glucose.

The presence of glucose in the blood triggers the pancreas to secrete insulin. Insulin is a hormone that attaches to the glucose and shuttles it into cells where the transformation into energy takes place. About eighty percent of the glucose you eat will get used right away as energy. The other twenty percent will be stored in the liver and muscles as glycogen, our storage form of glucose. A small portion of that twenty percent will also be converted into fat.

Between eating periods, it's the liver's job to make sure the level of sugar circulating in the blood doesn't drop too dramatically. Think of the liver as the control centre for blood sugar management. If blood sugar drops and no carbohydrate is available, the liver masterminds the release of various hormones and enzymes from various organs to free glycogen stores in an effort to bring it back up. If no glycogen is available, it orchestrates the creation of glucose from raw materials and stores found elsewhere in the body.

The ability of the liver and hormones to keep a steady supply of glucose flowing to your cells even when you don't eat is a marvellous example of the body's compensatory mechanisms that keep us safe. Unfortunately though, the perpetual influx of these hormones is also what can lead to all the negative effects associated with poor blood sugar management like those previously mentioned (i.e. overweight and obesity, depression, anxiety, moodiness, hyperactivity, aggression, sleep problems, poor appetite, sugar cravings, diabetes, hypertension, chronic infections, candida overgrowth, and likely a whole lot more).

So, let's look at this downstream damage caused by these hormones and how we can avoid it by eating for good blood sugar control.

PART TWO: Three Core Dietary Strategies for Raising Resilience

The most well-known effect of blood sugar imbalance is insulin resistance, which is a common contributor to weight gain and diabetes. Insulin resistance is less recognized for its contribution to heart disease, cancer, and hypertension, though these connections have been firmly established as well.

Insulin resistance is a condition in which the insulin receptor sites stop letting the insulin/glucose packages into cells. Glucose is locked out, remaining in the blood. The pancreas, dutifully doing its job, tries to lower that blood sugar by releasing more insulin. But because the cell's gatekeepers, the insulin receptors, are being way too selective about how much gets past, you end up with high levels of glucose and insulin in the blood, an exhausted pancreas, and not much energy being produced in the cell. The insulin also tells the body to store fat and it blocks the function of leptin, a hormone that tells your brain you're full. Therefore, insulin sensitivity causes increased hunger, reduced desire to exercise, and increased fat storage, i.e. overweight, moody, couch potato, sugar-craving kids. Certainly not the picture of resilience and health we imagine for our kids. While it used to take years to develop insulin resistance, we are seeing it more and more in children, largely because of dietary choices.

But there's more to the blood sugar story than weight gain, fatigue, moody behaviour, and diabetes (though of course those symptoms are very concerning). Remember, regulation of blood sugar is an intensively hormonal process masterminded by the liver. Those hormones can cause collateral damage as they try to carry out their blood sugar management duties.

The involvement of the stress hormones adrenaline and cortisol, on blood sugar is worth knowing about too. When blood sugar drops, adrenaline is one of the hormones the body calls on to release glycogen. We talked about adrenaline before when we talked about stress. Yes, adrenaline will release those glycogen stores but it also constricts blood vessels, dilates pupils, increases energy production, speeds up heart rate, and slows digestion. So, circulating adrenaline can look like a hyperactive, angry, aggressive, fidgety, distracted, irritable, and shaky child; symptoms easily mistaken for ADHD, but which actually can often be managed by regulating blood sugar.[67]

Children, it seems, release adrenaline sooner than adults do.[68] That is to say, a child's blood sugar does not need to be as low as an adult's before adrenaline is released. This makes symptoms of hypoglycemia (low blood sugar) sometimes more pronounced in children.

And what about cortisol? If the adrenal glands are continually called on to raise blood sugar level via adrenaline, they eventually call in the big guns, cortisol. Cortisol is like adrenaline on time release. It has some similar functions, yet works on a more long-term schedule. Like insulin, cortisol is thought of as a master hormone because it has such far-reaching influence. Cortisol exerts an influence on blood sugar metabolism, as well as on the function of the immune, nervous, and cardiovascular systems, and the regulation of systemic inflammation. Cortisol also adversely affects gut bacteria and can contribute to a digestive lining that is more permeable than it should be. It also slows the production of thyroid hormones. In this way, imbalances in cortisol (secondary to poor blood sugar control) can contribute to chronic infection, autoimmune conditions, weight gain, weight loss, heart palpitations, anxiety, moodiness, depression, sleeplessness, exhaustion, cravings, leaky gut, and constipation.

When you correct the blood sugar by changing how you eat, you influence these powerful hormones: insulin, adrenaline, and cortisol. You can see the far reaching consequences.

Because the brain requires real-time glucose for fuel (it cannot use stored glucose), the nervous system is the first to feel it when sugar is either consumed or unavailable. Most of us are familiar with that lightheaded, jittery feeling that signals the need to eat or the sugar high after eating sweets; this is the nervous system's response to sugar levels, high or low. Sugar's acute effects on the nervous system can also be felt as nervousness, irritability, anxiety, and headaches.

There is really no getting away from sweets. They will remain part of our life. With this in mind, understanding how sugar affects the body is important so we can make decisions about how and when to give it to our kids and take steps to mitigate the potential damage it can cause.

Why is Blood Sugar Erratic and What Can You Do About It?

There are a number of reasons a child might have a tendency towards poor blood sugar control, some of which are quite complex and beyond your control to manage. For example, they could have genetic issues with the release of insulin, or any other number of hormones or enzymes involved. They might have under or overactive adrenal glands, or a problem with their liver or thyroid. There are many contributors your endocrinologist can explain more completely, if needed.

However, let's focus on what we can control. Our most effective steps here are to choose carbohydrates wisely, maximize the nutrients needed for metabolizing carbohydrates, and shift eating patterns. We can also influence how the body manages blood sugar by addressing the biological stressors mentioned in Part One, like food sensitivities and yeast. You'll see how in a moment when I go through the twelve tips for blood sugar control.

Symptoms of Hypoglycemia (low blood sugar)
- high birth weight
- sleeplessness
- temper tantrums
- crying for no apparent reason
- hyperactive/overactive
- uncontrollable

- angry/hostile
- distractible
- Jekyll/Hyde behaviour
- headaches
- moody
- can't sit still
- cravings for sweets
- shaky/irritable before or after meals
- agitated
- defiant

Granted there are a variety of other contributors to these symptoms; however, if you notice your child displaying any of these, consider paying closer attention to their blood sugar stability. You might just discover a viable solution to help your child sooner than you might anticipate.

Before we get into the practical ways to control blood sugar fluctuations, let me turn to a common question I get about carbohydrates. What are you to do with a carboholic? Probably the most frequently expressed concern I hear from parents is that they can't get their kids to eat foods beyond those that are carbohydrate-rich (like white bread and pasta, candies, baked goods, and sweet fruit). I get it. Despite our best intentions and what we know about carbohydrates and sugar, the reality is that many kids crave it. When we talk about blood sugar management for children we need to keep this in mind, and keep it real. Those of you with carboholics might roll your eyes at some of these tips, muttering "ya, right" to yourself. I address carbohydrate cravings specifically starting on page 144, where you'll learn what drives these cravings and some very effective ways to break them. You'll then be able to come back to these tips here on how to keep carbohydrates in the diet in a way that supports stable blood sugar.

PART TWO: Three Core Dietary Strategies for Raising Resilience

Twelve Ways to Control Blood Sugar Fluctuations

1. Know Your Carbohydrate Sources and Choose Wisely
   Fruits, vegetables, dairy, grains, grain flour, and legumes have a higher concentration of carbohydrate and are, therefore, typically thought of as carb sources. In our western culture, the biggest sources of carbohydrates are grains and grain products, along with refined sugar. This includes baked goods, pasta, bread, whole grains, processed grains, and, of course, plain old sugar in its many forms.

   We used to categorize carbs as simple carbs and complex carbs, and were advised to avoid the simple and focus on the complex. Our understanding has since evolved, and the discussion now more commonly revolves around high glycemic carbs and low glycemic carbs.

   The glycemic rating of a carbohydrate refers to how quickly it gets broken down into glucose, prompting the release of insulin. High glycemic foods turn to glucose more quickly in the body and cause an insulin surge. Wheat flour, for example, has a high glycemic rating because the body easily and quickly converts those carbs to glucose. Blueberries, on the other hand, have a low glycemic rating because the type of complex carbohydrate in them converts more slowly to glucose. Low glycemic carbs are the type you want to focus on. They are like the slow burning logs on the fire, offering more sustained and reliable energy.

   Sources of Carbohydrates
   The best sources of carbohydrates are:
   - whole fruits that are low on the glycemic index: apples (particularly green apples), peaches, pears, plums, berries
   - starchy vegetables that are lower on the glycemic index:

Raising Resilience

sweet potato, carrot, celeriac, sunchoke, pumpkin, peas
- whole gluten-free grains, if tolerated: brown or wild rice, oatmeal, buckwheat, millet, quinoa, amaranth
- nuts: almonds, walnuts, hazelnuts, cashews, macadamia
- seeds: sesame, sunflower, flax, hemp, chia
- legumes and pulses and flours made from them: chick-pea, lentil, black beans, peas

Sources of carbs to offer in moderation:
Note: If you are seeing troubling symptoms related to blood sugar, you want to put these in the "carbs to avoid" group until you see improvement.
- fruits higher on the glycemic scale: pineapple, mango, ripe banana, dried fruit
- starchy vegetables higher on the glycemic scale: white potato, corn, parsnip
- gluten containing whole grains (and only if there is no sensitivity): rye, barley, spelt, Kamut, wheat
- fresh pressed fruit and vegetable juice
- whole sweeteners: Sucanat, honey, maple syrup, palm sugar
- low glycemic sweeteners: (see tip #8 in this section)

Sources of carbs to avoid:
These sources give you a burst of energy, but very little nutrition, and stress out the body.
- soda, including sports drinks
- refined white sugar
- refined white flours (bran removed)
- commercial fruit juice, even the "no sugar added" ones (see tip #6 in this section)
- low fat dairy (though it's often considered a protein source, it has a high concentration of carbohydrates as well, while providing few other helpful nutrients)

PART TWO: Three Core Dietary Strategies for Raising Resilience

2. Include Chromium-Rich Foods in Your Diet

   We don't need much of this micronutrient, but it is a critical player in glucose metabolism. Chromium helps insulin bind to insulin receptors, stimulating glucose transporters and helping to get glucose from the blood into cells. A lack of chromium can lead to insulin resistance and diabetes and all the associated health effects already discussed.

   Whole grains, green beans, broccoli, nuts, and egg yolk are good sources of chromium. Foods high in simple sugars are usually low in chromium and have been shown to actually promote chromium excretion.[69]

   Chromium uptake is increased when absorbed in conjunction with vitamin C.

3. Combine Macronutrients Wisely (fats, proteins, and carbs)

   Fibre, protein, and fat slow down the conversion of carbohydrate to sugar. When offering a child carbohydrate-rich food, consider what else is being offered at the same time. A piece of white bread from a loaf made mostly of white flour, yeast, and water is going to put more stress on the body than a piece of bread from a loaf made with more nutrient-dense flours like teff, buckwheat, or sorghum, along with eggs, flax seeds, and hemp seeds. The second is a better choice because it includes carbohydrates as well as protein, fat, and fibre.

   If you can't get your children to eat this more nutrient-dense type of bread, consider the snack as a whole. Accompanying that white bread with a bowl of raisins, orange slices, and fruit juice—all carbohydrate-rich foods high on the glycemic index—would be more stressful for the body than more nutrient-dense companions like nut butter, tuna, or a hard-boiled egg, which will slow down the metabolism of that white bread.

   You can use this same concept when you consider your meal planning. Take macaroni and cheese, a very carb-dense meal.

If your kids love it and look forward to it, consider how you might alter the meal for blood sugar control. You could use whole grain pasta that includes fibre, or a pasta made with a higher protein flour like buckwheat or quinoa or bean flour. You could add in butter, cream, or coconut milk for some healthy fat (refer back to the discussion on fats). You could serve some raw vegetables with it to increase fibre content. Or, if your kids will stand for none of these changes, you might pair your mac and cheese meal with a dessert that is high in fat and protein, like pumpkin custard made with coconut milk and eggs. As a whole, you've transformed this family favourite into a more blood sugar friendly version of itself, and boosted nutrient density at the same time.

Finding pleasing combinations of macronutrients will help slow down the metabolism of carbohydrates and reduce the stress on the body.

4. Incorporate Resistant Starch

Resistant starch is a particular kind of carbohydrate found in some starchy vegetables that resists normal digestion because we lack the appropriate enzymes to break it down.

Several studies have shown that resistant starch can improve insulin sensitivity in people with pre-diabetes,[70] and that it can lower blood sugar levels after meals.[71] One small study even showed that including resistant starch at breakfast can effectively manage glucose levels after lunch irrespective of the food eaten.[72]

Resistant starch is doubly supportive because it also has a positive effect on digestive health which in turn supports healthy blood sugar. We'll elaborate on this when we discuss digestion in the next section, Core Strategy #3.

PART TWO: Three Core Dietary Strategies for Raising Resilience

Some foods high in resistant starch:
- green plantains and green bananas: once they go yellow the starch is no longer of the resistant type. To retain their "resistance" to digestion, these should not be heated over 130 degrees. They are a nice addition to smoothies.
- cooked and cooled potatoes, grains, yams, and beans: the cooling process actually transforms the starch to become resistant (think potato salad, or mixed bean salad)
- raw potato starch and plaintain flour: use this in moderation; you can add it to smoothies or cooled soups
- Jerusalem artichokes (also called sunchokes)
- jicama

A word of caution, though; resistant starch is highly fermentable and it feeds gut bacteria. That's partly what makes it such an important part of a healthy diet. In most cases it has been shown to have a preference for feeding good bacteria, but if your child's digestive system is very unhealthy, you might find resistant starch will cause gas and bloating, and exacerbate symptoms of yeast. If this happens, you'll need to work on rebalancing digestive microbes before adding in resistant starch. Also, several studies have suggested that resistant starch benefits the body most when it is incorporated alongside other types of fibre in the form of a fibre-rich whole foods diet.

5. Focus on Breakfast
   Ensuring your child eats breakfast that includes some good fat, slow-digesting carbohydrates, protein, and fibre is the best way to stabilize blood sugar for the day. Try to get at least ten to fifteen grams of protein in a child for breakfast.

   Good breakfast ideas:
   - two eggs any style, cooked in coconut oil with chopped

spinach or other veggies with all-meal natural sausage, and apple slices
- oatmeal (not instant) with hemp, flax, and chia seeds
- berries with full-fat yogurt topped with flax oil and sunflower seeds
- homemade smoothie which should include some coconut milk or oil, some flax seeds, green vegetables, some berries, some hemp seeds, or Greek yogurt, or kefir (see Recipes for Resilience)
- French toast with whole grain bread and coconut milk cooked in coconut oil (see Recipes for Resilience)

Prepared breakfast cereals, breakfast bars, instant oatmeal, fruit juice, skim milk, flavoured yogurts, and frozen waffles tend to be harder on the body from a blood sugar standpoint. If you do need quick breakfasts, take a good look at the food label. Look for 12 to 15 g. of protein, at least 5 g. fibre, and no more than 8 to 10 g. sugar. Also consider what else you can add to your meal to balance it out, using your understanding of macronutrient combining as discussed in #3, above. A higher sugar breakfast like waffles and maple syrup would balance out with a high protein smoothie made with coconut milk and hemp protein, for example.

If you're having trouble getting breakfast into your older child, try a smoothie like the one in the Recipes for Resilience section. Or, if they really won't eat a thing, send them off with a nutrient-dense snack they can eat as soon as hunger sets in and before they get that hypoglycemic reaction.

6. Go Easy on Fruit and Juice

Barring certain medical or digestive concerns, having fruit every day is fine for a child who is otherwise healthy and growing well, as long as she is eating a whole, unprocessed fruit, with its fibre intact, like an apple instead of apple juice or a banana instead of a fruit bar. Whole fruit provides good fibre and micronutrients even though it is a source of sugar. The lower glycemic fruits like berries are easier on the body than the higher glycemic fruits like mangos and dates.

While a moderate amount of whole fruit is usually fine, fruit juice is best avoided as long as you can. Fruit juice contains about the same amount of sugar as an equivalent amount of soda pop. Really! 39 g. of sugar in a 12 oz. can of regular cola (9½ tsp), 31 g. sugar in 12 oz. of orange juice (just shy of 8 tsp), 39 g. sugar in 12 oz. of apple juice (almost 9½ tsp). Shocking, isn't it?

The type of sugar found in fruit juice is mainly fructose, which is not something we want to overdo in our diets. I've already mentioned that fructose can interfere with chromium, but there's more. Dr. Robert Lustig, Pediatric Endocrinologist at University of California, has become quite well known for his outspoken stance on the dangerous impact of fructose on the body, citing it as the major cause of diabetes and obesity.[73] Other research is confirming his theories that fructose is more toxic to the body than white sugar.[74]

Like glucose, fructose is a simple sugar. But it is metabolized a little differently than glucose. While all cells have the ability to metabolize glucose, the liver is the only organ with the correct transport mechanism to deal with fructose. Fructose does not stimulate insulin like glucose does. Instead, it gets transformed into fat by the liver, and leads to increased cholesterol, uric acid, and triglycerides. It can also lead to elevated blood pressure, insulin resistance, weight gain, and leptin resistance,[75] all issues that reduce overall resilience by placing undue burden on the body.

Again, for those of us with healthy metabolism we'd have to eat an awful lot of whole fruit in order to overdo the fructose. But when you add dried fruit, fruit leather, fruit juice, and high fructose corn syrup (HFCS) into the diet, levels increase quickly. The introduction of HFCS into the food supply has increased the average American's fructose consumption from about 15 g. a day (taken from fruit alone) to about 135 g. a day (with the introduction of processed food and beverages).[76] High fructose sweeteners, like agave, also have the potential to cause harm if eaten in large amounts.

There is no nutritional need for fruit juice. None at all. But if you do choose to keep it in your child's diet, here are some suggestions regarding juice:

- If giving fruit juice, water it down, using it more as flavouring.
- Go for quality when it comes to juice. Pay more and buy less, and think of it as a treat.
- Avoid drinking fruit juice with meals. It will fill up the tummy with empty calories, and leave less room for the more nutritious food you have prepared.
- Use juice to add flavour to smoothies and homemade jello, which also contain some protein (see the Recipes for Resilience section).
- Use fruit juice for homemade popsicles. Because popsicles take time to eat (more so than guzzling a glass of juice), your child will consume less juice while still enjoying some.
- Keep your juice consumption as a seasonal treat and delight in its flavour; fresh pressed apple juice during apple season is a good example. Just be aware of the blood sugar effect and don't overdo it.
- While it is true that fresh pressed homemade fruit and vegetable juice can be helpful for detoxification and can pack in the nutrients, take care to make sure your juice concoctions are not overloading your system with sugar.

PART TWO: Three Core Dietary Strategies for Raising Resilience

Water is the best beverage for a child. Herbal teas and fermented soda like kombucha or water kefir are next on my list. Avoid assuming your child needs juice.

7. Reduce Packaged Food

About half of the average North American's consumption of sugar is that which is added to packaged food. Reducing your reliance on packaged food is really the best way to cut down on sugar.

Once you start looking for it, you'll find added sugar in yogurt, teething biscuits, prepared baby foods, toothpaste, and cereals. The stuff is everywhere!

Some unlikely places you'll find sugar:
- sports drinks
- flavoured yogurt
- freezies and popsicles
- breakfast cereals
- teething biscuits
- baby foods
- granola bars
- bread

When you do purchase packaged foods, take a careful look at the label. Refer back to pages 41–42 for other names of sugar you might see on ingredients lists.

8. Choose Natural, Low Glycemic Sweeteners

I've already mentioned a few alternative sweeteners to try, but there are a number of wholesome, low glycemic sweeteners you can also use when you are cooking and baking, which will allow you to consume sweet things without causing metabolic chaos in the body. These sweeteners are also helpful if you are dealing with a yeast overgrowth, because most of them do not feed yeast the same way refined sugar does.

Here are some low glycemic sweeteners to try using:
- Green stevia leaf extract: you can get this as a powder to use in baking or in a liquid extract to sweeten beverages. It has a mild flavour that needs getting used to, but it has zero calories and does not affect blood sugar at all. It also has been shown to kill Lyme spirochetes.[77]
- Xylitol is a sugar alcohol the body can't fully digest or absorb. One study showed that xylitol can reduce acetaldehyde metabolites from Candida, so it can be helpful if you are battling yeast.[78] It is also known for fighting cavities. On the down side, it is typically grown on corn. For that reason, avoid it if corn is a problem for you, and if you do use it, get a type that is GMO free. Sugar alcohols like xylitol can cause diarrhea and general digestive upset for some people.
- Luo Han Guo is a sweetener derived from monk fruit. It has zero impact on blood sugar and is safe for those battling candida.
- Lakanto is a product that combines erythritol (a sugar alcohol like xylitol) with Luo Han Guo. It's a lovely low glycemic sweetener, but it is expensive.
- Yacon syrup is a bit like molasses syrup, and comes from the sap of the yacon tree. Its low glycemic rating is due to the high amount of inulin, which is a necessary food for probiotic bacteria in the digestive tract. Yacon syrup can cause gas in some people.
- Coconut nectar comes from the blossoms of the coconut tree. It has a low glycemic rating of 35, a mild taste, and is the consistency of honey (although it is less sweet).

Here again is a list of caloric sweeteners which, while they do impact blood sugar, are more nutrient-dense options because

they have their minerals intact and are lower on the glycemic index than refined white sugar.
- coconut sugar
- molasses
- Sucanat
- date sugar
- maple syrup
- honey
- apple sauce
- mashed banana

9. Reduce the Emphasis on Grains

   For years we have been told that the foundation of our diet should be plenty of whole grains. This is still the current recommendation of Health Canada's Food Pyramid. Certainly the fibre and micronutrients they provide are healthy and important, but within nutrition circles, grains, and foods derived from grains (like foods made with flour), have become somewhat of a contentious issue of late, due to their effect on blood sugar and digestive health.

   While grains can be part of a healthy diet, there are a few things to know about them.

   What you should know about grains:
   - We tend to eat too much of them, excessively increasing the carbohydrate content of our diets. Try removing them from your diet for a few days to realize how much you actually eat!
   - Most of the grains we eat are in their refined form (flour and flour based products like pasta, bread, pastries, and cereal). The more refined the grain is, the more vitamins, minerals, and fibre have been taken out or destroyed, and the higher its impact is on our blood sugar.

- Gluten, a protein found in some grains, is becoming more and more problematic. Gluten is often responsible for digestive discomfort such as IBS, bloating, and constipation, but we now know that about eighty percent of gluten-sensitive people have no digestive symptoms—the symptoms are neurological issues like headaches, ADHD, and depression.[79] Gluten sensitivity (or undiagnosed celiac disease) could be partly responsible for a child's hyperactivity, sleep disorder, attention issues, or learning problems. Gluten sensitivity has been implicated in over fifty-five conditions including autism spectrum disorders and increased risk of some cancers, obesity, schizophrenia, mood disorders, and osteoporosis.[80]
- If grains are going to be a staple part of the diet, it is best that they be properly prepared before cooking. Traditional cultures all knew that grains needed to be soaked and sprouted before being cooked and made into flour. Think traditional sourdough bread, for example. Here's why. There are compounds found in grains (also in nuts and seeds) that can wreak havoc on the body, causing inflammation and intestinal permeability.[81] Lectins have been shown to damage the digestive lining, and phytic acid has become known for its ability to pull nutrients such as calcium and zinc out of the body. Phytic acid and lectins are both somewhat deactivated by soaking and sprouting, however this process takes time and planning. It is also not typically employed in the process of making commercial ready-to eat-foods. Refer to the Nourishing Traditions cookbook[82] and Appendix D to learn how to prepare grains to reduce these anti-nutrients.
- Rice has been found to have high levels of arsenic in it so if you go gluten-free, make sure you're not relying solely on

PART TWO: Three Core Dietary Strategies for Raising Resilience

rice. Arsenic has been associated with the development of cancers in the skin, lung, bladder, kidneys, liver, and prostate, and might also contribute to diabetes, heart disease, and immune dysregulation. Consumer reports' testing suggests that the better choices are basmati rice from India, Pakistan, and California, and sushi rice from the US. These had the lowest levels of arsenic.[83] The same report found that rinsing your rice before cooking it also lowered the arsenic.

Whole non-gluten grains and pseudo-grains (like quinoa and amaranth) do have a place in the diet if there are no digestive or digestive-related health issues and if they are properly prepared and well tolerated. However, when looked at from a nutrient density or blood sugar standpoint, growing evidence suggests that grains should not be at the foundation of our diet. Try to get the majority of your family's carbohydrates from starchy and non-starchy vegetables and lower-sugar fruit. You may want to include some grains, but consider them carefully. We'll talk more about grains when we talk about digestive health.

10. Assess and Reduce Stress

You'll remember that one of the effects of the stress hormones cortisol and adrenaline, is to trigger the release of glycogen and raise blood sugar. When sugar levels drop due to, for example, forgetting to eat breakfast, this is a very appropriate response. But it's important to realize that when cortisol and adrenaline are released due to the activation of the stress response, like we talked about back in Part One, the same thing happens—a rise in blood sugar. Regardless of why the adrenal glands are called to release these hormones, they will still raise blood sugar. As you reduce stress you reduce stress hormones, which helps stabilize blood sugar metabolism. If you have a child who seems very reactive to sugar and carbohydrates, a good place to start is to consider their stress level.

11. Detect and Manage Food Sensitivities
The impact of undiagnosed food sensitivities will be discussed further in core principle #3 when we talk about digestion. I want to address it here as well though, because a sensitivity could lie at the root of your child's blood sugar control issues. Fundamentally, food sensitivity is an activation of the immune system in response to a trigger. An important by-product of this response is the inflammatory chemical, histamine. Histamine plays a role in metabolism, affecting blood sugar control, appetite, and fat deposition patterns.[84] So keep in mind that if you have tried all the strategies mentioned here to no avail, it might be excess histamine due to undiagnosed food sensitivities that is trumping your efforts to control blood sugar. We'll delve into more detail on detecting and managing food sensitivities in the next section.

12. Ensure Adequate Magnesium
Magnesium is needed for the secretion of insulin, which in turn is needed for the metabolism of sugar. Low levels of magnesium have also been shown to reduce the sensitivity of insulin receptors. While magnesium won't directly influence the up-and-down fluctuation of blood sugar, low levels might be a contributing factor to a child's blood sugar sensitivity and related symptoms. Here are some symptoms that might indicate a magnesium deficiency (see Appendix K for more):
- tremor
- agitation

PART TWO: Three Core Dietary Strategies for Raising Resilience

- depression
- cardiac arrhythmia
- potassium deficiency
- loss of appetite
- nausea
- vomiting
- fatigue and weakness
- numbness
- tingling
- muscle contractions
- cramps
- seizures
- sudden changes in behaviour

Sugar depletes the body of magnesium so if you have a sugar fanatic, consider supplementing with magnesium while you shift the diet. Some foods high in magnesium are: spinach, chard, pumpkin seeds, black beans, almonds, and avocados.

Section Summary

Feeding your family in a way that supports good blood sugar management supports resilience because it is a way to regulate hormonal balance. There are many dimensions to blood sugar control. Although not all, some of these factors are within your control to manage. If you're implementing all of these strategies and are still seeing signs you think are related to hypoglycemia, insulin resistance, or leptin resistance (refer to the list of symptoms mentioned), talk to your doctor about getting blood tests done and introducing some supplements and functional foods that can help support blood sugar metabolism.

Core Strategy #3: Support Digestion

Section Overview

Ensuring optimal digestive health has far-reaching effects on our general health. Good digestion allows us to effectively process and assimilate nutrients and eliminate waste. The digestive tract also serves as an interface between the internal and external environments, and much of our immune and neurological systems reside there. So digestive support is important if you want to strengthen the immune system or influence the brain.

Optimizing digestion has far-reaching effects on blood sugar, metabolism, energy production, inflammation, detoxification, immune function, mood, cognitive development, and even DNA expression. All of these elements in turn support resilience. As you've learned with respect to blood sugar and nutrient density, digestion also lies upstream of resilience. Taking steps to improve the health and function of the digestive tract is like greasing the gears of a bike; everything will run more smoothly.

Researchers are still unravelling the mysteries of digestive health, and will undoubtedly continue to discover much more about it in the near future. This section will help you assess the state of your child's digestion, explain what we do know at this point about why it is so important to protect, and give you steps to take to improve and nourish it. In addition, I've devoted an entire segment here to the digestion-allergy-asthma connection.

Keeping digestion on your radar and supporting it a little every day, as you'll learn to do in this section, will allow the body to do its job efficiently. And when it is thrown out of balance (which it will be), it will rebound quickly. If, however, symptoms persist despite implementing what we talk about here, working with a skilled practitioner on deeper digestive support is definitely your best next step.

PART TWO: Three Core Dietary Strategies for Raising Resilience

Understanding the Digestive System

Let's take a quick trip through the digestive process in order to understand how to best support it.

Digestion actually begins in the brain. Talking about food, smelling food, and yes, thinking about it starts chemical reactions in the body. (Perhaps this is why your kids run into the kitchen yelling for snacks right when you start cooking!) When we eat and chew our food, salivary amylase is secreted in the mouth which starts the process of carbohydrate digestion, turning the food into a mass called a bolus. The bolus passes down the esophagus and into the stomach.

The stomach is an acidic environment. The hydrochloric acid (HCL) in the stomach is essential for good health. Hydrochloric acid:

- destroys pathogenic bacteria, reducing the likelihood of food poisoning and infection
- transforms pepsinogen into its active form, pepsin, which starts the digestion of protein
- triggers the pancreas to release digestive enzymes into the small intestine
- triggers bile release from the gallbladder

Essentially, the stomach is where food is sanitized, protein digestion starts, enzymes are triggered, and certain nutrients like iron and B12 are prepared for absorption. Proper HCL level is essential for all of this to happen.

From there, the food mass passes into the small intestine, triggering the pancreas to secrete a host of enzymes to finish protein, fat, and carbohydrate digestion, and the gallbladder to release bile which emulsifies fat.

The surface area of the small intestine is immense. It is about twenty feet long, but it's folded into a sequence of peaks and valleys that dramatically increase the absorptive surface area. The peaks are also covered with little hairs, called microvilli, which increase the surface area even more. It's an immense organ.

The main activity in the small intestine is nutrient breakdown and absorption. It is here where digestive enzymes, perched at the end of the microvilli, finish the break-down of food into single molecule units you learned about earlier: amino acids, fatty acids, glucose molecules, vitamins, and minerals. These molecules pass through the cells of the intestinal lining and into the body where they are shuttled in various ways to cells for use.

By the time the food has passed through the maze of the small intestine, whatever is left continues on into the colon (also called large intestine) where it waits to be passed through the anus. The colon is teeming with bacteria. As stool waits here, water and electrolytes are absorbed into the body, and undigested carbohydrates are fermented into important fatty acids. The stool that passes out of the colon should be made up mostly of bacteria and fibre. Stool is also an important exit route for chemicals, hormones, and metals.

Think of the digestive tract as a long hollow tube, starting at the mouth and ending at the anus. It is actually considered to be external to the body, and its lining (which is actually only one cell thick) is an interface between the external and the internal environments.

The lining of the digestive tract hosts an army of immune cells. These immune cells patrol for anything passing through the lining they deem unsafe or foreign, along with any damage and inflammation. We'll come back to these immune cells when we talk about food allergy. It's recently been discovered that there's a very important nervous system living in the digestive lining. In fact, there are more neurons in the gut than there are in the brain. This so-called second brain we have is in constant conversation with the brain in our head, which explains why when we alter digestive function we also alter

PART TWO: Three Core Dietary Strategies for Raising Resilience

mood and behaviour (and might be why when we perceive fear or feel anxious, we feel it in our guts).

As you can see, digestion involves an interconnected web of factors including enzymes, bacteria, pH balance, and well-functioning organs and muscles. In order to properly digest food, all of these factors need to work in balance. A break down at any step can throw everything off.

We often think of the obvious when assessing digestive health—things like gas, bloating, constipation, diarrhea. But there are a whole host of symptoms that are digestive related but that you might not relate to poor digestion. For example, low stomach acid level can lead to B12 malabsorption, protein deficiency, and low iron, all of which can look like a child with poor energy and slower learning. That same HCL deficiency can muddle up the signal telling the pancreas to secrete enzymes resulting in poor carbohydrate digestion, which can look like a child with gas and bloating, but also poor growth and hypoglycemia. Poor bile production can lead to a fatty acid deficiency, which can look like a child who is spacey and gets sick a lot.

Does your child regularly experience any of the following?
- less than one bowel movement a day
- stool that is thin and watery
- stool that is sticky or greasy
- stool containing undigested food
- bowel movements that require straining, cause pain, or stink
- allergies
- eczema or patches of dry, scaly skin
- excessively smelly stool or gas
- yellow stool
- belly distention
- sugar cravings
- poor appetite

- burps, reflux
- cramps
- behaviour issues you can't get a handle on (e.g. temper tantrums, depression)
- headaches
- sleep troubles
- red cheeks and ears after eating
- chronic runny nose and cough
- recurring ear, sinus, or strep infections
- dark circles under the eyes
- excessive drool in children too old to drool
- lots of back arching (in babies)
- white coating on the tongue
- thrush
- unusual nail formation

If you answered yes to any of these questions, your child's digestion may not be optimal (and how's your own, by the way?).

You're not alone! The vast majority of children experience some of these symptoms. Does it really matter? Yes it does, if it persists. The body is a dynamic place, particularly the ecosystem of our gut. A short bout of diarrhea is not cause for concern, if it normalizes within a few days. The same goes for every one of the symptoms listed. But if several of these symptoms are persisting, it's time to take a close look at digestive function.

Because of the deep importance of nutrients, and because the immune and neurological systems are so highly influenced by what goes on in the gut, digestive care should be part of any health plan, no matter what symptoms are showing.

PART TWO: Three Core Dietary Strategies for Raising Resilience

What Causes Poor Digestion?
Remember back to what I said in Part One: we need to first remove what is counterproductive to make room for positive momentum. So what is counterproductive to good digestion in the first place? The following are some of the things that negatively impact digestive enzymes, microbial balance, and pH levels of the digestive tract:
- antibiotics
- certain medications
- chemicals
- stress hormones
- hormonal imbalances
- infections
- overcooked or processed food
- birth control pill
- birth by caesarean
- sugar
- cigarette smoke
- chlorinated water
- nonsteroidal anti-inflammatory drugs (NSAID), like Tylenol and Naproxen
- lack of certain nutrients
- steroids
- soft drinks
- heavy metals
- poor air quality
- yeast overgrowth
- parasites
- chlorine

It's not hard to create an imbalance in the ecosystem of the digestive tract. Our world has changed rapidly over the last sixty years, and so have our diets. Further, the digestive status of a mother is transferred to her baby. Certain parasites and candida yeast can pass through the placenta, and during labour the vaginal flora is transferred to our babies to kick start their microbial colonization. Our children are the second (perhaps third) generation to inherit dysbiosis caused by medications, pollution, stress, and poor diet. It has become more imperative than ever for parents of young children today to keep digestive health top of mind.

Supporting Digestion: The Role of Bacteria
Understanding the role of bacteria is key to understanding digestion. A healthy adult carries about 1.5 to 2 kg. (5 to 10 lb.) of bacteria, most of which resides in the large intestine (colon), yet also inhabits the small intestine, skin, nose, mouth, throat, lungs, and genitals. Here, we're going to focus on the microbes of our digestive tract.

The more we learn about these little bugs the more we appreciate their importance. Over thirty to fifty trillion microbes, including at least one thousand species of bacteria and yeasts, are involved in immune function, metabolism, digestion, detoxification, and DNA expression. They also seem to play a major role in regulating the pH of our digestive tract. This is why digestive support always involves some rebalancing of the gut bacteria, and why we should keep these little microorganisms at the forefront when it comes to health and resilience.

There are three families of bacteria living in our bodies: symbiotic, pathogenic, and commensal. To understand how they all work together, imagine a classroom of children.

The symbiotic bacteria are the goody-goodies of the class, the ones who do as they're asked, contribute only positive comments, run the student councils and clubs and are just a joy to have around.

The pathogenic bacteria are the colourful ones. They are the students who might have emotional baggage, and a temper. They keep their teachers on their toes, always learning. They push the teacher

PART TWO: Three Core Dietary Strategies for Raising Resilience

to become more creative and effective, however, if they aren't under careful watch, they can derail the teacher's efforts. In the body, the teacher is the immune system; the pathogenic bacteria (which really are only pathogenic if they get too strong) train the immune system.

The third group, the commensal bacteria, are the in-between ones. They are the highly influential kids who just want to fit in, and could go either way depending on the forces at play. If the symbiotic group in the class is strong, these folks will be pulled in that direction. If the pathogenic group is strong, they will be pulled that way.

In a healthy gut, the strength lies with the symbiotic group. The pathogenic group is only strong enough to keep the immune system in training but not enough to convert the commensal group.

Early childhood seems to be a programming period for our microbes. If we can set our kids up with positive microbial balance the body won't forget that information. If, on the other hand, a child has poor microbial balance, the body won't forget that either as the child moves through life. At this point (and our understanding is still evolving), researchers think that the microbial patterns set in childhood become a sort of set-point for later in life. Put another way, an adult who, as a child, had dysbiosis will have a harder time fixing the imbalance than one who started life with a well-balanced microbiome. This is why, when I work with parents who are starting to feed infants and babies, I focus a great deal on helping them support good microbial colonization.

Understanding and influencing microbes is at the forefront of medicine. They seem to carry within them an important key to unlocking the mystery of many health conditions including diabetes, allergy, depression, autism, multiple sclerosis, and obesity. The trouble is, while we are deepening our understanding of what microbes do in the body, there is still no consensus on how to go about fixing them when they are out of balance. Theories and strategies abound, but because everyone's gut profile is slightly unique, like a fingerprint, and because scientists are still mapping the microbiome and have not yet determined the perfect make-up, there remains a lot of trial and error when it comes to this part of digestive support.

I'm sure this will change in the near future, but for now the only thing most researchers seem to agree on is that robust microbial diversity is good for your health, while disease is associated with diminished diversity. The nine suggestions I outline in this section are tools and strategies that support the many components of the digestive system, including the microbes, and that I have seen improve resilience.

The Allergy-Asthma-Digestion Connection
The rate of food allergies in children has risen dramatically over the last decade. As of 2014, it was estimated that one in thirteen children had a food allergy.[85] The National Institute of Health estimates that one in twenty children under the age of five have a food allergy.[86] A 2012 health survey found 4.1 million children has food allergies.[87] In terms of sensitivities, estimates as high as one in four have been made. Parents are terrified of certain foods, more and more kids are carrying epinephrine injectors, and we're seeing good nutritious foods being banned from school lunches. Asthma is also on the rise, affecting an estimated 334 million people worldwide. Because it is also an immune-related condition that can be helped by supporting digestion, I'm including asthma in the discussion here.[88]

In Part One, you learned about four ways allergies and sensitivities can be a barrier to resilience. There is a strong connection between these conditions and digestion, so implementing the tools in this section will be very helpful for those of you managing allergies. I want to spend some time addressing this.

Before diving deeper into the allergy-asthma-digestion connection, let's first distinguish between a sensitivity, an allergy, and asthma.

PART TWO: Three Core Dietary Strategies for Raising Resilience

Allergies, sensitivities, and asthma are all conditions that involve the immune system. In an allergy, immunoglobulin type-E (IgE) antibodies of the immune system attack what they see as foreign (the peanut protein, for example). The IgE antibody attaches itself to the allergen and activates the release of a variety of chemicals, including histamine. The symptoms of an allergic reaction result, typically occurring within minutes or hours of the allergen entering the body. Doctors make a diagnosis by testing for the presence of IgE antibodies in the blood and anti-histamines are often used to manage symptoms. Anaphylaxis is a severe IgE reaction in which massive amounts of inflammatory chemicals are released throughout the body, causing constriction of the airway and a drop in blood pressure to the extent that life is threatened.

Sensitivity is the term given when symptoms are found but the IgE antibodies are not. In this case, other antibodies of the immune system, such as IgA, IgG, and IgM are being mobilized, while IgE are not. There is still an immune response triggered and inflammation is initiated, yet the antibodies being mobilized are not detected by a typical allergy test because the test is not looking for them.

Symptoms of a particular sensitivity can take up to four days to appear after the trigger enters the body, and can range from changes in mood and energy to headaches and digestive issues. Over two hundred symptoms have been associated with food sensitivities. Some of the most common are listed in Appendix E.

Sensitivities account for about ninety percent of adverse reactions to food; they are extremely common and often go undiagnosed.

In both cases—allergy and sensitivity—the immune system is being mobilized by the presence of an antigen (or trigger) resulting in the release of inflammatory chemicals.

Asthma is similar, in that it also involves the hyper-stimulation of the immune system leading to symptoms. In the case of asthma, symptoms manifest in the respiratory tract. Many children who have allergies often progress to asthma in a process called "The Atopic March." This term explains the common progression of immune hyper-sensitivity that starts with dermatitis, moves into allergy, and then to asthma.

I mentioned in Part One how allergies present a barrier to resilience. The inflammation involved can contribute to all kinds of health conditions like eczema, celiac disease, Crohn's disease, paediatric depression, ADHD, headaches and migraines, and diabetes; the persistent release of chemicals like leukotrienes, histamine, and serotonin, further throw the body out of balance. Some medical research suspects that allergies signal the initial stages of more complex autoimmune diseases.[89]

What's the connection with digestion and how can you help your asthmatic or allergic child with this core strategy? As it turns out, research is now showing that digestive health is closely related to immune function, which makes good digestive care a key strategy you can use for preventing and resolving food reactions and asthma (along with all the other health conditions associated with inflammation and immune activation that have been previously mentioned).[90]

You'll recall that just inside the gut lining lays a border patrol of immune cells. They are there to protect the internal environment of the body from invaders. Antibodies are the soldiers of the immune system. There are slightly different types of patrols (IgM, IgG, IgE etc.). While charged with a few varied tasks, they are all looking for compounds they determine are not in the appropriate place. When one is detected, they attack and destroy it; then stimulate inflammatory chemicals (like histamine) and create antibodies to prepare for the next time that offender comes around.

With a sensitivity or allergy to food, the question to ask is, *Why is the immune system mounting an attack to a food instead of allowing it to pass by patrols and nourish the body like it's supposed to?* The problem is not the food, it's the body's response to the food.

PART TWO: Three Core Dietary Strategies for Raising Resilience

Part of the answer is that people with allergies tend to lack certain immune cells called T-regulatory cells (T-regs), the absence or malfunctioning of which allows the immune army to run amok, much like a ship without a captain. This was the conclusion of researchers who studied the immunological difference in groups of children before and after they grew out of their dairy allergy. The difference was in the T-regs. There might be a genetic explanation for poor T-reg function but it also seems that nutrient deficiency may play a role. We can bolster their function by ensuring good nutrition is coming in (use the tools you learned in Core Strategy #1) along with ensuring good absorption by focusing on the tools I give you here.[91]

A second part of the answer is that when food is not sufficiently broken down, the immune system of the digestive tract fails to recognize it. You'll remember that the process of digestion is supposed to break foods down into glucose, amino acids, and fatty acids, which, along with vitamins and minerals, are allowed through the digestive lining to be used by the body for growth and function. This digestive process should effectively transform all food into particles the body recognizes thereby rendering all food hypoallergenic. But in some people it doesn't, which results in inflammation and irritation of the gut lining and the initiation of an immune system response. This is why, when it comes to allergy and sensitivity, keeping the offending food out of the diet is only part of the solution. Improving digestive capacity, fortifying the gut lining, and nourishing the immune system is the other part of the equation. In fact, promising research has been done to show that changing gut microbes in infants can significantly reduce the likelihood of developing allergy and asthma.

Can Probiotics Prevent Allergy?

The Swansea Baby Allergy Prevention Trial is one study that investigated the safety and efficacy of probiotic bacteria in the development of allergy. Four hundred and fifty-four mother-infant pairs participated in the double-blind placebo trial. The study group was given a daily dose of four strains of probiotics from thirty-six weeks gestation through infancy up to age six months. The children were assessed for adverse reaction, atopic eczema, and allergy at six months and then again after two years.

In terms of safety, the results showed no adverse events were caused or exacerbated by the probiotics. In terms of efficacy, while they did not see a significant immediate reduction in eczema in the infants, they did find a fifty-four percent reduction of allergy to cow's milk, eggs, grass pollen, tree pollen, house dust mites, nuts, and fish, when tested at two years old, as measured by a skin prick test.

Various other studies have shown a decrease in nasal congestion and watery eyes provoked by environmental allergy to grass, dust mites, and pollen. The probiotic test strains which included various forms of lactobacillus bacteria sometimes worked better than antihistamine and improved quality of life substantially.

All of this emerging research gives great promise to the use of probiotics in the prevention and treatment of allergies by altering the microbial environment of infants. If you're going to try probiotics for allergy relief, continue for a minimum of six weeks before deciding if you've seen an effect. If you're going to use it for your infant in attempts to prevent allergies, use a probiotic that has been formulated for infants and has been well tested.[92]

Detecting Food Allergy
Diagnosing an allergy is quite straightforward. You would be referred to an allergist who would do a skin prick test and/or a blood test to determine if IgE antibodies are activated in response to an antigen. If there is a response, there is an allergy. You will typically be instructed to remove that antigen from the child's life as much as possible. Periodically, the blood would be retested for antibodies and, if they are low enough, your doctor might recommend re-exposure.

Diagnosing a food sensitivity is more difficult because testing is unreliable and expensive. You can get an IgG food panel done, to test for the presence of IgG antibodies to hundreds of different potential food allergens. You can also test for IgA antibodies. Food sensitivity testing like these can give you a starting point for understanding which foods are causing problems and some good insight into where digestion might be breaking down.

The most reliable test for food sensitivity is an elimination diet:

1. Take out the most likely allergens for a minimum of three weeks (along with anything revealed in any IgE or IgG testing you've had done) and look for changes in symptoms.
2. You then reintroduce each food individually, waiting four days between introductions, and look for symptoms. The presence of a symptom indicates a food sensitivity.

The elimination diet is very helpful, yet can often be a difficult and subjective tool. There are also several different versions of it. Appendix G outlines in more detail how I suggest you conduct this diet if you suspect food sensitivities.

This diet will give you direction as to which trigger foods might be a problem for your child. Adapting your diet accordingly will take a burden off of the immune system; that food will no longer be counterproductive to your efforts of raising resilience. After that, to actually build resilience, the focus should turn to supporting the digestion process as outlined in this chapter, as well as on improving nutrient density as detailed in Core Strategy #1. If digestion is well supported and the immune system is properly nourished, you should be able to eventually reintroduce some of the offending foods.

QUICK NOTE
Do not reintroduce foods to which your child has an anaphylactic reaction until your doctor has tested their antibodies and given you the go-ahead.

Why Not Just Rely on Medication for Allergies?

Steroids and antihistamines are the medications typically prescribed for allergies. In the case of an anaphylactic-type allergy, self-injectable epinephrine (also called adrenalin) will also be used. Steroids and antihistamines effectively reduce the symptoms like increased mucous, watery eyes, and itchy skin by blocking the action of mast cells and eosinophils (the cells that mediate the allergic response). Epinephrine is used in the case of anaphylaxis to rapidly reduce bronchial swelling and stabilize blood pressure, followed by antihistamine to suppress the release of histamine.

Certainly, the occasional use of these medications can help with your quality of life and in the case of anaphylaxis ALWAYS have access to epinephrine and antihistamine until your doctor gives you the all-clear. But none of these medications address the underlying cause of your symptoms.

Your child's allergies and asthma are a call to action. Follow the Raising Resilience plan by reducing stressors and implementing all three of the core strategies (particularly #1 and #3) to help support the natural health and regulation of the immune system.

Nine Ways to Support Your Child's Digestion

1. Strategically Introduce Foods
   If your child is between six to twelve months old, I highly recommend that you follow my guidelines in the Thriving Babies course to introduce solid foods. You can find details about it on my website, at www.JessSherman.com. Inspired by the Gut and Psychology Syndrome digestive-healing protocol, along with elimination diet principles, the Thriving Babies course teaches parents how to start with highly nourishing, yet easier-to-digest foods that are supportive of digestion and beneficial for babies. This is helpful for all babies, particularly for those who were

PART TWO: Three Core Dietary Strategies for Raising Resilience

born via Caesarian section (C-section), given antibiotics early in life (or during birth), fed formula, or showed early signs of food or breastmilk sensitivity.

Babies born via C-section have different gut bacteria at birth than those born vaginally.[93] This is likely why C-section babies have a higher chance of developing asthma and celiac disease.[94] Protecting digestion by being careful how you introduce foods can reduce that chance.

Further, this approach of strategically and methodically introducing new foods can help if you've detected that any of your family has sensitivities. This way you can tell quickly whether certain foods will be well tolerated, or best not to serve (at least until you're able to determine the root cause).

2. Set a Calm Tone for Meals (and Generally Reduce Stress)

I know this one can be tricky for busy families, but making sure your child sits and focusses on enjoying his food instead of eating while multitasking (reading, watching TV, playing video games) or walking around, can help digestion a great deal by reducing stress hormones.

When you relieve tension, slow down, and focus, you improve digestion by activating the parasympathetic nervous system which prompts the release of the "rest, digest, and grow" hormones. Anxiety and worry, and eating on the run, activates the sympathetic system which shunts resources away from long-term priorities like immune function and digestion.

Also, cortisol can cause inflammation of the gut lining, and seems to have the ability to open up the tight junctions of the gut and lead to increased intestinal permeability.[95] It can also destroy beneficial gut flora.[96]

To improve digestion, try concentrating your energy on making eating sessions peaceful to allow the parasympathetic nervous system to do its job and generally reducing stress. Furthermore, take some time after your meal to remain in that restful mode so that digestion can finish. This can be hard (or impossible) when you have to rush off to a soccer practice, but understand that if you don't find a way to factor in this time, you might experience some digestive consequences. A game of cards, reading a story, or working on homework would be more restful.

3. Include Probiotic Supplements (and/or Fermented Food)
   Include some sort of fermented food in your child's diet. A properly fermented food is one that is high in the type of bacteria, and sometimes healthy yeast that keeps the gut environment in a healthy balance. Remember that I included bacteria as an essential micronutrient due to its role as one of the master regulators of the body. Also recall that a healthy gut has about 5 to 10 lb. of bacteria living in it, whose jobs range from digesting food to regulating immune function and metabolism, but that there are myriad ways they get disturbed. Including fermented food in your child's diet is the best way to keep the inner ecosystem of the gut healthy.

   Good quality yogurt and kefir are the easiest to incorporate, as long as your child can tolerate dairy. It takes about thirty seconds to make your own kefir and yogurt, and the advantage is you can be certain the fermentation time is a full twenty-four hours which breaks down the troublesome proteins and sugars in the milk (casein and lactose) and ensures the enzymes and microbes are strong. If purchasing fermented dairy, take a close look at the list of ingredients and choose one free of fillers, gums, or pectins; these are added to thicken yogurt that has not been properly fermented or has had its fat taken out. For yogurt choose one that has only whole milk and bacteria as ingredients. If buying kefir, choose one that is made in the traditional way, with kefir grains, and contains no added sugar. Use yogurt and kefir to make smoothies, popsicles, mix with fruit, or use in salad dressings and baking (baking will kill some of the bacteria, but the process of fermentation has still rendered it more digestible).

Sauerkraut, kimchi, kombucha, and water kefir are other options, if you are a little more daring. They're not as hard as you may think to make, and are very, very helpful as well.

I encourage all families to experiment with simple home fermentation, and they are always pleasantly surprised at how quick and easy it is to do!

If you just can't get fermented foods into your child, you can supplement with a good quality probiotic. Using fermented food is more helpful than a probiotic supplement because it helps correct stomach acid and pH levels of the digestive tract, brings in prebiotic fibre to feed the probiotic bacteria, and increases the variety of microbes and enzymes.

But a good quality probiotic is the next best thing. You'll likely want one that has a combination of lactobacilli and bifidum strains, and it's best to alternate brands every so often so as to diversify the species. Remember that there are about 1,000 different species in the gut. We need them all to be present and strong. Microbial diversity is a key to good health. You'll not get that much from a supplement, but it's a start.

I want to include one caveat regarding fermented food. Fermented food might not be a helpful choice if your child has a strong case of candida yeast overgrowth, small intestinal bacterial overgrowth, or histamine intolerance. You'll know ferments are not a good idea for your child if they react with bloating, abdominal pain, or worsening symptoms of yeast and dysbiosis (as described in Appendix M). If that happens, go with a low dose probiotic supplement, increasing steadily as tolerated, and periodically try small amounts of fermented food until tolerated.

The use of fermented food to correct dysbiosis is a rather controversial topic among health practitioners. I have found that while most people can reintroduce them eventually, if pathogenic bacteria have a stronghold on your gut, fermented foods can be too strong at the start of treatment.

Avoiding chlorinated water, household and environmental chemicals, and the other items listed on page 113 that interfere with digestive microbes, is equally important for maintaining microbial diversity.

4. Include Broth Made From Animal Bones
Homemade broth made from animal bones has come out on top as the best food for nourishing and repairing a damaged gut lining in most people. The nutrients, primarily the gelatin, glutamine, and minerals found in broth are particularly healing for the gut mucosa. It's also a great source of easy-to-digest amino acids, particularly glycine which can be lacking in the diet because animal muscle meat typically has fairly low levels.

The broth you get in tetra packs or cans is NOT the same thing as what you make in your kitchen from scratch. That type of broth offers flavour but little nutritional value. It's easy to make wholesome homemade broth, even with a busy schedule; and it's one of the most cost-effective tools you have for improving your child's health. Directions for making this can be found in the Recipes for Resilience section at the back of this book.

Obviously this strategy won't work for vegetarian families. Homemade vegetable broth is a great way to get added minerals into the diet, and you'll find a recipe for it in the Recipes for Resilience section. But vegetable broth does not offer the same healing properties as broth made from animal bones. There is

PART TWO: Three Core Dietary Strategies for Raising Resilience

no comparable vegetarian source of the healing gelatin and gut-supportive nutrients you get from broth.

5. Include Foods Known to Heal, Soothe, and Nourish
There are many foods which help to heal, soothe, and nourish the gut lining, stimulate digestive juices, and reduce inflammation. For example:
- Garlic and onions stimulate the production of bile which is needed for fat digestion.
- Lemon, raw apple cider vinegar, and fermented vegetables will help normalize stomach acid levels and general pH of the intestinal tract.
- Peppermint, ginger, raspberry leaf, and chamomile teas are soothing and toning to the stomach lining.
- Papaya and pineapple contain protein-digesting enzymes.
- Okra, leeks, mushroom, slippery elm, and licorice root can be helpful for healing a damaged lining.
- Foods high in vitamin D, A, essential fatty acids, and zinc will nourish the digestive lining (see Appendix A for food sources).
- Some foods shown to decrease inflammation in the body include berries (particularly blueberries), turmeric, ginger, wild fish (salmon or sardines are good choices), cold-pressed unheated virgin olive oil, cruciferous vegetables (like broccoli or kale), garlic, and green tea (the tea is good for you, not your kids!)

You'll find many of these foods incorporated in the Recipes for Resilience section.

6. Ensure Proper Elimination (i.e. Relieve Constipation)
We can't talk about digestion without talking about poo (okay, elimination).

Raising Resilience

How many parents have you talked to who are struggling with this; relieving constipation in their youngster? It's so common that it has become normal. But it's not normal. It's a sign of poor digestion, and it's critical to relieve it.

Poor elimination reduces resilience in two ways: by blocking one of the body's methods of flushing toxins (the stool), and by generating more toxins as stool sits in the colon.

Have you ever noticed that when a child has to poo their behaviour changes? Now you know why.

Here are a few contributors to constipation:
- stress
- food intolerance
- lack of fibre
- too much fibre
- sugar (can also cause diarrhea)
- dairy (in some children)
- lack of good bacteria
- insufficient stomach acid
- poor fat digestion (problems with the liver or with bile)
- parasites
- dehydration

What to do:
- Vitamin C (ascorbic acid) is a natural laxative and improves the production of HCL in the stomach (further enhancing digestion). Using an ascorbic acid supplement can relieve constipation (choose one that is not buffered and can be mixed with water to get the added benefit of hydration). Avoid using this for a prolonged period; just use it as needed to relieve the body while you try to identify the underlying cause of the constipation. Start with 1000 mg. and move up until stools soften. Stop if your child feels any other side effects.

PART TWO: Three Core Dietary Strategies for Raising Resilience

- Magnesium is also a natural laxative. It can be given as a supplement starting with the following doses and increasing until stools soften: 1 to 3 years 65 mg. per day; 4 to 8 years 110 mg. per day; 9 to 18 years 350 mg. per day. There is little risk of taking too much magnesium, but if your child feels any symptoms other than soft stools, stop. And if there is diarrhea, cut back.
- Think zinc. Zinc helps trigger digestive enzymes and gets digestion moving. I like using a liquid as it is particularly easy to give to children and is highly absorbable. You can also get zinc as a lozenge. The risk of zinc overdose is possible, so you don't want to use high doses without consulting a practitioner, but if used as directed and for a short time it is quite safe to try for constipation relief.
- Increase probiotics, as they have been shown to relieve constipation (and diarrhea). There is, as of this point, no toxic upper limit for probiotics. If your child experiences mood, digestive, or skin reactions to a probiotic, cut back. Try to work up to twenty billion CFUs per day. Stubborn cases might need more than that, however, you should consult with a practitioner first.
- Assess for food sensitivities. If a child is eating food he is not digesting well, his gut will be inflamed and irritated. This can lead to constipation. See Appendix E and G for more details about how to detect food sensitivity.
- Assess stress. As discussed, stress hormones will cause digestive issues like constipation because they effectively shut down the digestive process. Go back to Part One to identify and relieve stressors.
- Increase dietary fat and decrease protein. Fat tends to lubricate whereas protein tends to bind. Coconut oil is particularly helpful because it does not require bile to be digested

like most fats do. Those who are constipated can sometimes lack bile. Olive oil and flax oil can also be helpful, though start by increasing coconut oil.
- Include lemon, ginger, and apple cider vinegar in the diet to help support healthy hydrochloric acid levels.
- Rub castor oil on the abdomen in a clockwise direction around the belly button. Do this several times a day.
- Consider a digestive enzyme to help the body break down foods better.

Remember, constipation has a root cause. You just have to find it. If none of these strategies are working, find someone to work with who can help you dig deeper.

7. Avoid Gluten (and Go Easy on Grains)
As we already discussed in the context of blood sugar, grains are hard to digest. They contain phytic acid and lectin (and sometimes gluten), which all interfere with nutrient absorption, and they do not offer the best nutrition for a child.

Let's dive into a bit of the research on gluten and lectin in particular, as they relate to digestion.

Lectins are proteins that bind to carbohydrates. They are found in all foods. There are two subcategories of lectins that are sometimes called toxic lectins because they are so hard to digest and can interfere with digestion. The two subcategories are called prolamins and agglutinins. Gluten is a type of prolamin.

Prolamins and agglutinins are found abundantly in the seeds of grasses (grains and pseudo-grains like wheat, barley, corn, rye, spelt, Kamut, amaranth, quinoa, and chia) and legumes (like peas, beans, peanuts). We are not good at digesting prolamins and agglutinins; we lack the proper enzymes. A vital

PART TWO: Three Core Dietary Strategies for Raising Resilience

body will compensate for the lack of enzymes by drawing on certain bacteria in the gut to do the job instead. So unless the gut bacteria are in tip-top shape (and we already went through the myriad reasons why they might not be), lectins are left undigested and cause irritation and inflammation to the gut lining.

Gluten seems to be particularly problematic. Gluten, you'll remember, is a type of protein found in some grains. Being a prolamin, we lack the enzymes needed to pull gluten chains apart into single amino acids, forcing our gut bacteria to do the job. Gluten also seems to be able to simulate the production of zonulin, in some people, particularly if digestive microbes are not up to snuff. Zonulin is a protein that regulates the opening and closing of the tight junctions between cells of the intestinal lining. An overproduction of zonulin is associated with leaky gut, inflammation, and autoimmune disease.

So, all this to say, if digestion is not optimally balanced (as it is not in many of us), gluten and other lectins may actively interfere with digestive health. This is partly why many nutritionists will advise that you adopt a gluten or grain-free diet while trying to improve your digestion.

We're continually learning about the effect of lectins on the body, and it's still quite early to completely pass judgment on these foods. But given that they have the potential to exacerbate leaky gut, burden the gut bacteria, and stimulate the immune system, I caution parents to approach foods high in toxic lectin with moderation and caution.

A child with strong digestion and immune function can likely handle some foods that are high in toxic lectin. But basing a diet around them I think is a mistake. Long term, it is likely to wear down the body's compensatory mechanisms. I generally advocate for a diet that avoids the gluten grains, and includes moderate amounts of gluten-free pseudo-grains and legumes. If

Raising Resilience

you are actively trying to repair the gut or immune function, I think it wise to cut these foods out altogether for a period of time. Once digestion is vital and strong, you can introduce them again if you wish.

8. Focus on Flavonoid-Rich Foods

    Flavonoids are phytochemicals; they are natural chemicals found in plants, and are considered a micronutrient essential for health. Phytochemicals were discussed in Core Strategy #1.

    Flavonoids are found in fresh fruits and vegetables, particularly those that have a rich colour. Red grapes, blueberries, blackberries, citrus (though be careful as lots of kids are sensitive to citrus), purple potatoes, onions, and purple cabbage are some foods rich in flavonoids. They seem to have a protective effect on the tight junctions in our digestive lining, reduce gut inflammation, and help regulate probiotic bacteria colonies.[97]

    When foods are stored, cooked, and processed, flavonoid content is dramatically decreased.[98] So eating some raw foods and the freshest possible, including a rainbow of colours, will help ensure good flavonoid intake.

    A word of caution. Flavonoids are a member of the phenol family. Some children, particularly those with conditions associated with very imbalanced gut microbes like autoimmune disease and autism, might not process phenols very well and they can become counterproductive to the goal of raising resilience. Refer back to Part One, page 52 and Appendix J for common symptoms of phenol sensitivity. If your child has a phenol sensitivity, this particular strategy will not be helpful for improving digestive health until you uproot that sensitivity. For the vast majority of children, though, phenols are a very healthy, even essential, part of the diet.

PART TWO: Three Core Dietary Strategies for Raising Resilience

9. Add More Fabulous Fibre

Adequate fibre in the diet is critical for optimal digestive function. Fibre nourishes gut bacteria, creates important fatty acids, bulks up stool, speeds up the passage rate through the digestive tract, and helps to eliminate toxic compounds.

You already met resistant starch—a particular form of fibre that is helpful for blood sugar regulation. Because it is so highly fermentable, resistant starch is particularly helpful for digestion; it feeds the healthy microbes down there and initiates the process of fermentation which creates a short chain of fatty acids including butyrate which is a primary energy source for the cells of the colon. Resistant starch in the diet has been associated with reduced incidence of leaky gut and cancer.[99]

Refer back to page 97 for food sources of resistant starch, but keep in mind that all types of fibre are important to digestive health. Include whole foods like beans, pumpkin, cauliflower, nuts, coconut, seeds, and high fibre fruits like apples and apricots every single day. Most of us don't get nearly enough fibre in our diets. Start to pay attention to how much your child is getting by reading food labels. If you think it's less than about 20 g. a day, consider adding a fibre supplement to mix into foods and drinks to support digestive health. Choose one that combines both soluble and insoluble types of fibre.

Increase dietary fibre slowly as it can be irritating to a damaged digestive tract. If you see evidence of gas, bloat, pain, constipation, or diarrhea you need to either move more slowly or hold off on this strategy while you work on the others. Then try again.

Part Two Summary

36 Ways to Help Your Child Relax, Learn, and Grow

15 Ways to Maximize Nutrient Density
1. Incorporate Healthy Fats into Your Cooking
2. Avoid All Trans Fats
3. Learn to Ferment Your Own Foods
4. Try Cooking with Seaweed
5. Super-Enrich Your Grains
6. Try Nutritive Teas
7. Use Hemp Seeds
8. Join a Community Supported Agriculture (CSA) Group and Visit Local Farmers' Markets
9. Join a Food-Co-op (Buying Club)
10. Reduce Sugar and Swap Out Your Sweeteners
11. Swap the Salt
12. Boost Veggie Intake
13. Swap Out the Flours
14. Invest in Good Kitchen Equipment
15. Incorporated Targeted Quality Supplementation

12 Ways to Control Blood Sugar Fluctuations
1. Know Your Carbohydrate Sources and Choose Wisely
2. Include Chromium-rich Foods in Your Diet (whole-grains, broccoli, nuts.)
3. Combine Macronutrients Wisely (fats, proteins, and carbs)
4. Incorporate Resistant Starch
5. Focus on Breakfast
6. Go Easy on Fruit and Juice
7. Reduce Packaged Food
8. Choose Natural, Low-glycemic Sweeteners

PART TWO: Three Core Dietary Strategies for Raising Resilience

9. Reduce the Emphasis on Grains
10. Assess and Reduce Stress
11. Detect and Manage Food Sensitivities
12. Ensure Adequate Magnesium

9 Ways to Support Your Child's Digestion
1. Strategically Introduce Foods
2. Set a Calm Tone for Meals (and Generally Reduce Stress)
3. Include Probiotic Supplements (and/or Fermented Food)
4. Include Broth Made from Animal Bones
5. Includes Foods Known to Heal, Soothe, and Nourish
6. Ensure Proper Elimination (i.e. Relieve Constipation)
7. Avoid Gluten (and Go Easy on Grains)
8. Focus on Flavonoid-Rich Foods
9. Add More Fabulous Fibre

PART THREE

SELF-REGULATION AND ENVIRONMENT

Section Overview

At this point you've learned about the major stressors that interfere with resilience and three core strategies to focus on to support it. In this section we layer on one more consideration: food environment, where we address how we eat. You've perhaps noticed that our children learn as much, perhaps more, from their environment than from what we say with our words. They absorb everything that surrounds them. They're influenced by routines, clutter, colours, and they copy our mannerisms and body language. They are little sponges.

So far we've talked about how what we eat can be a powerful tool for building resilience, but in this section we'll look at ways to cultivate a positive relationship with food by attending to how we eat. I'll explain how that helps build physical resilience, and share some common pitfalls that can be counterproductive. There is also an entire section here devoted to managing picky eaters.

Positive Food Relationships

When I give workshops, I ask parents this question: *Envision your child fifteen to twenty years from now. Imagine they are living on their own for the first time. What do you want for your child in terms of their association with food?*

Think about this for a minute.

What generally emerges from this conversation is some version of the following; we want our children to:
- eat for hunger, rather than for emotional reasons
- stop eating when they're full and not overeat

Raising Resilience

- make healthy food choices at the grocery store
- try new foods and be adventurous
- know how to select and prepare a diversity of healthy foods
- have good table manners

Thinking of the bigger picture and reverse engineering can help you keep calm and focused when you find yourself engaged in a battle over broccoli with your seven-year-old.

Eating Competence is a term coined by dietitian Ellyn Satter, a true pioneer in the field of feeding children. The image described above is the profile of what Ms. Satter would term a competent eater.[100]

A competent eater is a person who:

- eats when they're hungry, stops when they're full
- can determine when they're eating for emotional reasons and when they're actually hungry
- can make good judgements about what to eat
- has good table manners
- eats foods they like because they want to, not because they have cravings or aversions
- learns to be open to, and like new foods
- is accepting of foods that help them grow

Eating competence supports resilience, and it's not difficult to see how. Indeed, research on competent eaters has shown them to have better Body Mass Index (BMI) profiles,[101] healthier physical self-acceptance,[102] they are more active,[103] sleep better,[104] eat more nutritious diets.[105] They are even at a lower risk for several chronic diseases including heart disease. Competent eaters are more physiologically and mentally resilient. Longer term studies have also shown that competent eaters are more likely to pass on competent eating

PART THREE: Self-Regulation and Environment

to their own children, thus extending all the benefits to the next generation.[106]

How do we raise a competent eater? How do we promote a positive relationship between our kids and their food? Satter has been involved in, and has compiled vast research showing that how we eat as families, and the environment in which our kids eat, has as much or more of an impact on our health than what we eat does, because of its impact on our eating competence. Paying close attention to how we talk about and approach food, as well as to what our expectations are around food and eating will be our strategies here.

I've used some of Ms Satter's techniques in my own nutrition practice, and through trial and error have added some of my own based on her research. Here are five strategies I teach my clients that help them foster a positive relationship with food and develop eating competence.

Five Tips for Fostering a Positive Relationship with Food

1. Provide Structured Meal and Snack Times
   Most children do well with a breakfast, mid-morning snack, lunch, mid-afternoon snack, and dinner. This type of pattern keeps blood sugar stable and provides consistent nutrients for the growing body. From a food competence perspective, the regularity and predictability of adequate food also helps your child understand that his hunger needs will be met, while cutting down on your work load. Consistency helps children become familiar with their hunger and satiety cues and, ultimately, learn to eat appropriate amounts throughout the day. As you shift your meals and snacks to ones that are more nutrient-dense too, you'll find that your children will naturally fall into a healthier eating pattern, even reducing their needs for handouts.

I find that sticking to a predictable structure is particularly helpful for children who struggle with anxiety or blood sugar instability, even if it might feel counterintuitive at first. We already talked about how stress hormones affect behaviour and appetite. Providing structure brings predictability, reduces stress, discourages eating on-the-run or multitasking while eating, promotes good digestion, and teaches your children that eating and drinking are to be done sitting down and with focus. Be sure to provide enough food at meal/snack times so they can feel full and sustained until the next eating time. Later, we'll also talk about how this can be a powerful strategy to manage picky eaters.

2. Eat Together and With Intention

    Eat meals sitting down, and as a family whenever possible. This helps fosters connection and attachment. Research has shown that children who engage in family meals at least twice a week with at least one parent, enjoy better academic success, have less substance abuse, experience fewer depressive symptoms, and are less likely to smoke.[107] This has less to do with what our kids eat and more to do with how they eat.

    Exactly why this is remains unclear. Maybe because of the connection we foster over meals, maybe because they are benefiting from reduced stress. Regardless, eating together brings significant health benefits. Try to make the atmosphere as calm as possible. Having a routine can help such as lighting candles, saying grace, having a moment of silence, or setting/decorating the table. Eat with your kids and have them eat the same foods as you. Resist the temptation of becoming a short order chef or having your kids eat meals at a different time from you.

PART THREE: Self-Regulation and Environment

3. Don't Forsake the Taste
   Food is nourishment but it should be enjoyed too. Use the strategies you've learned in this book to make meals and snacks that are nutrient-dense and appealing for your child. If you insist they eat foods that taste like cardboard (though they might be nutritious) they will start to look elsewhere for food handouts (friends, corner store, etc.). Learn to make nutrient-dense, simple, delicious meals, and snacks from whole, real foods like the ones at the back of this book and on my website.

4. Mind Your Language and be Open to Exploration
   Talk to your kids about food in a positive way. Remark on colours, textures, flavours; talk about where it came from, try new varieties; and try to meet farmers—make eating an adventure. There are approximately one thousand varieties of bananas in the world,[108] about twenty-five species of cultivated carrots,[109] And about four thousand varieties of potatoes.[110] Can you imagine the number of edible plants and animals that exist on this planet? While it might appear that we have a lot of choice at the grocery store, try keeping track of exactly how many different foods you actually purchase and eat. You'll likely be surprised at the limited number in your repertoire. Is it perhaps about twenty? Explore food with your children. They like to be given choices, and will often eat more if they see you explore new things.

   Variety is particularly important for toddlers, as they are developing their palettes. They are quite literally learning what to expect the flavour of food to be. Offering a variety of real, whole foods with different colours, textures, and shapes helps train children that this is what food looks and tastes like. If we feed them a bland diet of processed foods early on, they are likely to come to expect that type of diet in the future. After about age three, most children become what is called neophobic, wary of new things. Offer lots of variety early on. Be patient with their pickiness, and keep offering.

Some ideas to improve the adventure and increase variety:
- Bring home unfamiliar foods from the store or market and taste them together; look them up on the internet and find out about them together.
- Meet local farmers, find out what they're growing, and how to cook and serve it.
- Try new ethnic recipes that might offer different flavours from what you're used to.
- TIP: When offering a new food/flavour, make sure there are also some familiar foods on the table, just in case the new ones are not appreciated initially. You want to encourage your kids to be honest about their likes and dislikes and not be scared of new foods—encourage them to try it, they don't have to like it or finish it. But you don't want them to go hungry if they didn't like it.
- Decorate your table with several options of side dishes like chopped veggies, avocado, or sauerkraut. Your child is likely to eat more if she has a perceived choice.
- Start a backyard garden and sow both familiar and new plant varieties you've never heard of before.

5. Trust. And Allow Your Children to Learn to Self-Regulate
Resilience, in its essence, is the ability to self-regulate; what we are doing when we raise resilience is supporting the body's innate mechanisms for self-regulation. When it comes to food choices, hunger, and satiety, we can again learn to listen to the body's wisdom. Healthy babies know when they are hungry; they know when they are full. Healthy children and toddlers know what they like and what they don't like.

PART THREE: Self-Regulation and Environment

It is totally normal for a young child to:
- like a food one day and hate it the next
- eat everything in sight one day and nothing the next
- be wary of new, unfamiliar foods

Unfortunately, starting at a very early age, factors come into play which interfere with our ability to self-regulate. We talked about some of them in Part One and cover a few of them in this section as well. When these get in the way, many of us have to reconnect with our natural hunger rhythms as adults.

It takes a great deal of trust and faith that a child will learn to accept new foods without coercion, but studies show that most will, if given the opportunity.[111] Reducing stressors (Part One) and implementing the three core strategies (Part Two) is going to significantly enhance your child's ability to self-regulate. I have seen this time and again. At the end of this section I'll go through some instances that might require some extra help beyond these tips. But to start with, here are a few ways help your kids learn how to self-regulate around food.

- Instead of insisting they finish everything or coaxing them to eat more, allow them to leave food on their plate if they are full. But no snacks should be given right after the meal; they need to learn to know what full feels like, and be honest.
- Allow them to taste a food and decide they don't like it ... that day. Then try it again a few days later. It sometimes takes twenty or even thirty tries before a child will accept a new food. Keep at it and experiment with preparing it different ways.
- If you need a reward system, use stickers; or celebrate with a game instead of using sweets.
- Instead of talking about certain foods as bad or banning foods, teach your kids about moderation. Use

everything you've learned in this book about the impact of food on the body to help them make connections between what they eat and how they feel.
- Be enthusiastic about the colour, smell, texture, and taste of ALL foods, not just (but including) sweet foods or desserts (and encourage grandparents to do the same).
- Avoid falling into the "he won't eat that" trap and creating too many alternatives for your child. Keep offering. Keep modelling. Keep trying.
- Allow your child to have some choice at meal time and, as they get older, talk to them about how to make positive choices.
- When it comes to dessert, incorporate a nutrient-dense dessert into the meal instead of holding it ransom.

Now, if you've tried all of this—and I mean you have been super consistent with these strategies for at least a year—yet you're still struggling with eating competence and food relationship, read on, and let's talk about picky eaters and special circumstances.

Managing Picky Eaters

When I talk with parents about these concepts of eating competence and food environment, we invariably end up in a troubleshooting discussion about picky eating. What do you do when you understand nutrient density, you know which foods are best to support your child's physiology, you understand the core principles and the concepts of self-regulation and eating competence, and you've even figured out how to make time for all this in your busy schedule, yet you can't get your kids to really eat the way you want them to?

Truth is, change is hard. Implementing all the information in this book is not going to happen overnight. In Part Four of *Raising Resilience*, I lay out a road map to help you make the transition, but

PART THREE: Self-Regulation and Environment

first, let's turn to the issue of picky eating for some ways to understand it and strategies to manage it.

Picky eaters come in all forms. You get the ones who don't want to eat anything or just want to eat white bread and pasta; there are those who are hooked on junk food, or others who will eat everything one day and nothing the next. Then you get some who will eat foods as long as they aren't mixed with (or touching) other foods.

Picky eating is often blown off as either a stage, or perfectly normal, or as something he/she will grow out of. I disagree with this categorical approach, and believe pickiness is something that needs managing. We need to actively teach our kids to become competent and confident eaters, just like we actively teach them to tie their shoes and pick up after themselves. Some children don't need as much coaching on this; it's enough to just model good behaviour, offer good food and follow the suggestions I've already laid out in this section—but picky eaters do need our attention. As with all behaviours and symptoms, there is a root issue when it comes to picky eating. Something is driving their behaviour and it presents a very serious roadblock in your efforts to raise resilience. Fortunately, we can turn to the Three Core Dietary Strategies to help us determine contributing factors and uproot picky eating from the inside.

Nutrient Deficiencies and Picky Eating

Your picky eater might have some particular nutrient deficiencies and benefit from supplementation. There are certain nutrients that are associated with the hormones that regulate hunger, satiety, and the senses of taste and smell. If a child is deficient in these, then her internal cues might be off.

Zinc, B12, and B1 are the nutrients that have been most well researched in relation to taste, appetite, and hunger. Vitamin C, iron, and the rest of the B vitamins might also be at play. Blood tests can confirm any deficiencies but, generally, a fairly short trial of about three months of supplementation will tell you if this is going to help. If you want to try some experiments, I suggest you choose one at a time.

How to assess if nutrient deficiencies might be part of the picky eating problem:

- Take a look at your child's fingernails. Little white spots can indicate mineral deficiencies, particularly zinc. If you see that your picky child has a lot of these, this nutritional support might be just the fix you need.
- Is your picky child also exhausted? This is a common sign of B12 deficiency.
- Is your child a vegetarian or refusing meat? Zinc and B12 might be low, exacerbating the pickiness. Assess if there are other sources of these nutrients in the diet.
- Does your child avoid protein such as meat? She might have low stomach acid and therefore have difficulty digesting protein, making her feel uncomfortable. Try extra Vitamin C and zinc which help boost hydrochloric acid secretion. If she has low stomach acid, she could also be low in iron and B12 which are prepared for digestion in the stomach.
- Does your child's immune system seem sluggish? He gets sick all the time and has a hard time getting over colds? Vitamin C and zinc might be low, contributing to the picky eating behaviour.
- Has your child been diagnosed as anemic? Look at iron, B12, and folic acid levels. Also assess stomach acid.
- Was your child breastfed? If so, what was the mother's mineral status while breastfeeding? If she was depleted, it's likely her breast milk was too.
- Does your child also suffer from constipation or diarrhea? This could indicate malabsorption and low B12.

Picky eating can throw kids into a vicious cycle of nutrient deficiency. They are lacking in certain nutrients; their hormones and taste buds get thrown off; they develop food aversions; they become more deficient. In this case, good quality supplements can be a great help to interrupt the cycle and resolve the picky eating.

Blood Sugar and Picky Eating

Blood sugar imbalance can also cause picky eating, particularly in the form of carbohydrate cravings. Your body knows that eating carbohydrates is the quickest way to raise blood sugar, so when sugar drops, carb cravings ensue. Refer back to Core Dietary Strategy #2 for a refresher on why that is, plus other approaches you can take to support healthy blood sugar levels. Often, once blood sugar is regulated, carbohydrate cravings subside and a child is more willing to try new foods. I find attending to blood sugar helps particularly well with children who are picky as well as hyperactive, moody, or lethargic.

Digestive Insufficiency and Picky Eating

It could be that your child's pickiness is not simple preference; it is a physiological craving brought about by an imbalanced gut ecosystem. Sugar feeds yeast and bacteria, so when those are proliferating in the gut, they call out for more and more. They want to be fed. What this looks like on the outside is a carbohydrate addiction, i.e. the child who only wants to eat plain pasta, white bread, and crackers. The child craves and eats sugar, the yeast and bacteria proliferate, leading to more intense sugar cravings.

The way to break the cycle of carbohydrate craving caused by dysbiosis is to feed the good bacteria and knock back the pathogenic bacteria and yeast. Probiotics and fermented foods are essential and, sometimes, if it's well-established dysbiosis, an antifungal is needed, (Sporanox, olive leaf extract, or grapefruit seed extract, for example). It will depend on your child and you'll likely need some help with this. When the gut is rebalanced, the pickiness often subsides.

Gluten and dairy are particularly addictive foods when they are not digested well by a person who has dysbiosis. With this perfect storm in place, the peptides in the gut create compounds that connect with opioid receptors in the brain and can act like a drug. These kids are severely addicted and it is often not a pleasant experience to help them break free (though it will make them healthier in the long run!)[112]

How to assess if digestion might be part of the picky eating problem:
- Does your picky eater have a history of antibiotic use, frequent infections, developmental delays, chronic constipation, or diarrhea, skin rashes, allergies, colic, or reflux? If so, correcting digestion might be the route you need to take to break the picky eating behaviour.
- Does your picky eater have any of these classic symptoms of yeast overgrowth: violent behaviour, inappropriate laughter, hyperactivity, looking drunk, tummy aches, bloated belly, bedwetting, inattentiveness, anger, and aggression, high-pitched squealing, athlete's foot, or persistent diaper rash?

If you want a more solid diagnosis about what's going on in the gut, a comprehensive stool analysis or organic acid test can be ordered. These will show certain metabolites present in the urine or stool that indicate which yeast or bacteria are proliferating. Your nutritionist or naturopath can order them.

Three More Tips for Managing Picky Eaters
While implementing the Three Core Dietary Strategies might resolve your picky-eating situation, there are a number of social contributors to this behaviour as well.

Your child might be testing boundaries and trying to exert control. That's what kids do. Part of the art of parenting is creating a safe space for exploration that also has strong, predictable boundaries. It's easier

PART THREE: Self-Regulation and Environment

said than done, I know, but to further help, here are three ways to help your picky eater expand her boundaries.

1. Avoid Making Food a Battleground

Battling about food, even a little, is likely to escalate and become a major issue. It's particularly important when dealing with picky eaters that you remain calm, relaxed, controlled, and tell it like it is.

Food is one, and maybe the only place a child has some real control, some leverage. They just have to close their mouths and there's nothing anyone can do about it. The bonus for them is that it throws you into a tailspin of a reaction. That's some serious leverage!

Let me tell you now and save you the heartache; you won't win this one. You'll just get all worked up.

What you can do is provide good food. Let me say that again—provide *good food*—not cater to his every whim and not let him decide what good food is.

I caution you against becoming the short order cook. This can get out of control really quickly and can put unwanted stress on your already busy schedule. Not only is this short-term solution hard on the parent, but it passes a level of decision-making about what healthy food is, on to a child who isn't ready for that yet.

Before you can allow your child to make decisions about what constitutes a nutritious meal, you have to be certain he or she knows a little something about nutrition. So gauge that for yourself and incorporate their suggestions gradually.

TRY THIS ...
- If your child refuses to eat what is provided, that's okay. Still, do your best to get him to sit at the table with the family.
- Parents, remind each other that your job is to provide nourishing food, and your child's job is to put it in his mouth and swallow it. This kind of division of labour comes from Ellen Satter who has used it successfully for decades.[113] I have

also found that keeping the line dividing these responsibilities distinct and not crossing it helps a great deal.

Examples of crossing the line:
- letting your child choose what's for dinner, unless they are older and know a little something about good nutrition
- forcing your child to sit until the plate is clean
- telling your child she needs to eat a few more bites
- telling your child he is not full when he says he is

Don't force, bribe (more on this shortly), scream, hold food or toys ransom, or punish. It's really important to remain calm and just tell it like it is. For example, say: "This is our meal; take what you like and say, 'No, thank you,' to what you don't like."

Don't get me wrong; your child might actually be hungry and say she's not. But my point is that it's not up to you to tell her she is hungry. She is finding the boundaries. She is learning. She is going through a process. You can ask questions like, "Are you sure your belly is full?" However, she needs to remain in control of the phrase, "I am full." Make it clear, though, that there will be no more eating after the meal is over. Let the learning happen. She will be better for it in the long run.

2. Positive Reinforcement

There is a very subtle yet big difference between bribery and positive reinforcement.

Bribery means you hold something ransom. "You get such-and-such if you do such-and-such," or "You will have such-and-such taken away if you don't do such-and-such." With bribery you do something if they do something. Positive reinforcement is rewarding the behaviour you want to see more of once they have done it. It uses the concept of earning, and gives them the reward only after they have done

PART THREE: Self-Regulation and Environment

what's expected. Positive reinforcement shines the spotlight on positive behaviour.

An example of positive reinforcement is a sticker chart: you earn a sticker after we see the expected behaviour; perhaps five stickers earn a bigger gift. Verbal praise, simple as it is, might also work well. Gossiping about your child's good behaviour to someone else, knowing they are within hearing distance, is probably my favourite positive reinforcement tool. In a sly effort to make them feel proud of themselves you say to your spouse something like, "Wow, Sophie tried carrots today. I'm so proud of her!"

The behaviour you want to reinforce will depend on your situation. You can incentivize good behaviour at the table, or reinforce trying a new food. You may even want to use this to encourage your child to put a food to his lips, or take a bite even if he spits it out. It will depend on the level of pickiness you are dealing with.

Now, three important caveats with using positive reinforcement to manage picky eating:

a) Avoid focusing on the amount of food that is consumed. Instead, reward your child for pushing their boundaries. Reward positive behaviour that you want to see more of.

b) Avoid using foods as your reward of choice. If you make dessert, it is part of the dinner and everyone is entitled to some, not just those who behaved in a certain way.
TIP! It helps a great deal to make your desserts nutritious, which is something I always recommend anyway. Pumpkin custard, rice pudding, and apple crisp are some of my favourites. Make an extra effort to have a nourishing dessert on days when you're trying out a new recipe that you're not sure everyone will like.

c) Your love for them is unconditional, and special time together is important. Avoid bringing your relationship into the mix by using special time together as an incentive.

I hope I have made clear the difference between bribery and positive reinforcement. While they might seem similar, they send different messages. Positive reinforcement works very well as an incentive for picky eaters; it puts the spotlight on positive behaviour and encourages them to do more of it. Be cautious, though, and remember the big picture. Ultimately, you want your children to be self-motivated to eat when they are hungry and stop when they are full, but as they learn to do that, you can use this technique to reward their willingness to push boundaries and try new things.

3. Consistency

Most kids love consistency. Having a predictable routine around food makes them feel comfortable. We've already outlined how consistency around eating helps reduce stress, reduce your work load, and develop eating competence.

It might feel counterintuitive to restrict eating to certain times and places, but I find it actually helps resolve picky eating. Try to think big-picture again. By being consistent you are ultimately teaching your child to feel secure and comfortable around food and feeding. If anxiety is part of the picky eating, a consistent pattern that your child can come to rely on will be beneficial.

Grazing, like bribery, can spiral out of control very quickly, and I caution against it, though please keep in mind that I'm talking about children over the age of about two here. Children under two typically have more irregular eating patterns, and that's okay.

TRY THIS ...

Offer breakfast, lunch, and dinner, and have mid-morning and mid-afternoon snacks. You might want to throw in a snack before bedtime too. That's it. Avoid handouts at other times. Of course, sometimes the schedule will get a bit screwed up on busy days, but the more you stick to this schedule, the better things roll. The pickier your child is, the stricter I suggest you be with consistency.

PART THREE: Self-Regulation and Environment

Make sure to have enough food at each eating time so that your child can eat her fill. Try to have something new and something familiar and include a combination of healthy fats, proteins, and low glycemic carbohydrates as you learned to do in Part Two. Use positive reinforcement when your child tries a new food. Remember that you are attempting to build trust and confidence.

Your child might be grouchy about this shift at first. This is new and different. This is taking away some of their control (control that I suggest should be yours at first anyway). It might seem as though it is backfiring as your child exerts his control by shutting his mouth. Stick to the plan.

Solving your picky-eating problem will likely involve a combination of all of these strategies. Implement them one by one; starting with whichever you feel is the easiest to wrap your head around. Be patient. Your child is learning a lot of things all at the same time. So are you. Be supportive and encouraging. Be a good model.

QUICK NOTES:
When to be concerned about a picky eater (and seek some help):
- Their pickiness is sustained for a long time and you start to worry about nutrient intake.
- They are avoiding whole food categories (protein or carbohydrates, for example). This might indicate a digestive problem.
- They are severely craving certain foods. This might indicate a food sensitivity or digestive imbalance.
- They are gaining or losing excessive weight.
- A breastfed baby starts to refuse her mother's milk (before age appropriate weaning).

When to be concerned about an overeater (and seek assistance):
- They always want to indulge in sweets or carbohydrates and won't eat anything else.

- Their growth pattern does not follow the curve that is optimal for them. Please note, some children are larger than others; what matters most is that they are following a curve rather than following a pattern of peaks and valleys.
- Their eating pattern is also accompanied by other troubling symptoms like sleep apnea, fatigue, lack of motivation, depression, anxiety, or excessive weight gain.

The Influence of Sensory Misreading and Poor Oral Motor Skills
Some children might be having difficulty learning how to manage their tongue, chew, and swallow. If they can't effectively do those things, then they likely won't want to eat much or might be very selective about textures.

This situation calls for a referral by your doctor to a speech therapist or occupational therapist with oral-motor training and experience releasing retained reflexes.

Section Summary
Fostering eating competence and creating a positive food environment in your home has far-reaching effects on physical resilience. Research shows that, if left to their own devices, most healthy children will eat enough nutrients and calories to sustain their optimal growth pattern. A child who is forced to eat (i.e. "You can't leave the table until your plate is clean") is likely to eat less and become picky; a child whose food is restricted ("Don't eat that; you've had enough and it will make you fat") is likely to eat more than they need and become overweight.

That said, other research has shown there are a few underlying factors that can get in the way of this natural tendency to self-regulate that may need to be addressed if your efforts don't seem to be yielding results. Refer back to the discussion about picky eaters and the QUICK NOTES about when to find help.

PART THREE: Self-Regulation and Environment

When we learn to respect their likes, dislikes, hunger, and satiety cues, and gently help them to push their boundaries and correct underlying confounding factors, we encourage our children to become competent eaters, all the while trusting it will work out in the end. This has both a direct and indirect impact on their physical resilience and overall wellbeing. This delicate balancing act which we are responsible for can ultimately help us raise healthy, responsible young people who will in turn teach their children the wisdom of competent eating.

PART FOUR

Transitioning to Resilience: Finding Your 80/20

Raising healthy kids is top of mind for most of us, but let's pause for a second, and consider something supremely important. I learned early on in my mothering career, and also in my nutrition career, that any discussion about a child's health is not complete without also addressing the health of their caregivers. Here's the thing, we simply can't raise happy, healthy kids if we aren't happy, healthy parents. We can only raise resilience if we also support our own health and sanity. In order to do that, we have to make realistic goals, stay organized as much as we can, and find the wiggle room.

If you're feeling overwhelmed and confused about where to start, then stop, and take a deep breath. This section will guide you through the process of transition.

The 80/20 Rule

We've talked in this book about how factors like sugar and additives interfere with resilience and also of how focusing on the three core strategies—maximizing nutrient density, regulating blood sugar, and supporting digestion—improves your child's resilience. You now know more than some doctors about how food affects the body, and you have some very concrete strategies to implement at home. However, when the reality of our busy lives sets in, we may not be able to, or want to, spend all our time in the kitchen. We are faced with

Raising Resilience

daily choices at the fridge, stove, and grocery store. We want to do the best we can with the time and money we have, and I know many of us tend to be hard on ourselves when we pick less healthy options. "I don't even want to know!" some parents tell me. Indeed, sometimes it's hard when you know what you should do, yet find yourself in a position where you either can't or don't want to. It's a little easier on the conscience to plead ignorance. But now you can't do that because you *do* know (and I know you want to know, or you wouldn't have gotten this far in the book).

So here's the thing, we will not nail all of this all of the time. None of us will. Your child will be exposed to all those forces that interfere with resilience from Part One. They will eat blue birthday cake at a friend's house, likely take a course or two of antibiotics, eat chemical-laden popsicles at a soccer match, and breathe polluted air. They will get bent out of shape more than once, but that's why the concept of resilience is so powerful. By sharpening your skills of observation and implementing as many of these strategies as often as possible, you can support the body's strategic ability to bring itself back into balance when it is thrown off course. Your resilient child will rebound quickly and efficiently when you drop the ball, so you can stop stressing about it.

I call this "finding our 80/20." It's a spin on the Pareto principle, also called the 80/20 rule. In economics, the Pareto principle is mostly used to explain how inputs and outputs are generally not in balance; that twenty percent of your efforts will yield eighty percent of your results. The core principles for raising resilience are an application of the Pareto principle, in that simple changes yield massive results. As it applies to the day-to-day feeding of your family, though, there's a slight shift in emphasis; while these changes might be simple, you must be mindful of sticking to those changes eighty percent of the time if you want to see results.

PART FOUR: Transitioning to Resilience: Finding Your 80/20

These numbers, 80/20, are arbitrary; it's the concept I want you to embrace. The concept is that because of the body's phenomenal mechanisms for keeping itself in balance, and its desire to be resilient, if we can support it with these simple changes most of the time, it can usually take up the slack. The healthier your child is, the more slack it can take up.

Note one caveat here. There are certain medical conditions that cause a breakdown in the body's compensatory mechanisms and require some careful dietary consideration. Celiac disease requires that gluten be eliminated from the diet. Anaphylactic reaction to peanuts requires the complete elimination of peanuts. Type 1 diabetes requires careful control of dietary carbohydrates. These kinds of issues are not part of the 80/20. They are absolutes. The body is unable to compensate, and we must take steps so that it isn't asked to. There are even severe sensitivities which, despite the lack of an official diagnosis, lead to such dramatic symptoms that they become absolutes. For example, the elimination of casein might become an absolute if it improves eczema. And the elimination of gluten might become an absolute if it triggers migraines. You might have discovered some of these types of sensitivities already, or maybe you will if you follow an elimination diet as described in Appendix G. Those absolutes aside, you get to decide which of the strategies outlined in this book give you the most bang for your buck, which are essential to focus on, and what are within your ability to apply. In a moment I'll help you figure that out.

First, here are a few examples from my nutrition practice to illustrate how the 80/20 principle can apply:

Debbie came to me because her four-year-old son was experiencing severe constipation. He was also experiencing an eczema-like rash that just wasn't getting better. Understandably, he was irritable and uncomfortable and his behaviour was often difficult to manage.

Raising Resilience

By trial and error, Debbie and I deduced that a major contributor to the constipation was dairy. When we relieved the constipation by removing dairy and adding in some micronutrients (i.e. we removed a stressor and improved nutrient density), he was better able to concentrate, tantrums lessened, and appetite increased. The severity of his rash also decreased once bowel movements improved.

When we added fish oil, probiotics, coconut oil, and ghee to the diet, (i.e. we further increased nutrient density and added in some digestive support) her son's temperament became less erratic and his sleep improved.

For Debbie's son, an optimal diet is dairy-free, with lots of quality fat. These simple dietary measures did not require massive changes in effort, but certainly brought huge changes in his happiness, health, and function. This became the core of Debbie's feeding strategy and she sticks to it eighty percent of the time or better.

Now if her son eats dairy on occasion, or if she forgets the supplements, she knows he is likely to have a few off days, although now she has strategies to quickly get him back on track. Of course, the more she sticks to his ideal diet, the more she can allow for some flexibility periodically.

Here's another example:

Stella's seven-year-old autistic daughter's inability to concentrate at school, along with her lack of impulse control, were causing growing problems. We deduced that gluten, certain dairy products, food colouring and, to a lesser extent, foods high in phenols, were triggers that seemed to make her behaviours worse. Keeping gluten and food colouring out of her child's diet became absolutes for Stella because it had a dramatic effect on her daughter's wellbeing. She kept the dairy and high phenol fruit out most of the time, but discovered some wiggle room there.

Stella's daughter was a vegetarian, so I was concerned about certain nutrient deficiencies. We tried fish oil supplements, which helped

PART FOUR: Transitioning to Resilience: Finding Your 80/20

improve her focus. The family agreed to include more fish, grass-fed meat, and fish oil, along with a few other supplements to support her digestion and detoxification. We continued to make dietary modifications until we had a strategy that helped her function at her best.

Stella and I devised a very particular ideal diet based on what we learned by watching her daughter's reaction to certain foods. She identified her absolutes (food colouring, gluten, and non-fermented dairy), and then found her wiggle room (high phenol fruits and yogurt).

This is how transformative nutrition can be when you match dietary strategy to individual physiology. But as you can see, different children, diverse physiology, different ideal diets, diverse 80/20.

Knowing how certain foods affect your child's particular physiology, and using that to create your 80/20, helps you become more efficient at making food decisions. This allows you to confidently relax and take the stress out of feeding your family.

Your Plan For Transformation

Now that you've read the whole book (or at least the summaries), have a broader perspective on how to raise resilience, and you've learned about all the strategies you can use, here is a plan for moving forward.

First, I suggest you make the following two lists:

List #1 contains what you are already doing well. List all your triumphs and acknowledge your accomplishments.

- Are you already using some of the supplements suggested?
- Have you already nailed the positive food environment?
- Have you already focused on nutrient density?

Of the things we've covered in this book, what are you doing well?

Raising Resilience

List #2 consists of your health goals, for you and for your kids. This list has to do with the vision you have for your family's health. What would you like to see happen?
- More energy?
- Better focus?
- Better sleep?
- Reduced allergies?
- Fewer tantrums?
- Fewer sick days and a more efficient immune system?

What are your main struggles and what would you like to see change? Be as specific as you can. You will refer back to this as you move through your transformation.

Consider this. The transition to resilience requires a new way of thinking. It's a lifestyle shift and it takes time. Some of you might be chomping at the bit to shift everything right away, particularly if your child is struggling. But for most of you, it's not realistic to do so. You have a busy, full life and that is not going to change overnight. You need to find time and space for this and your family needs to adapt to these changes too. So instead of thinking of raising resilience as a linear path, taking you from point A to point B in a short amount of time, I suggest you think of this as a circular strategy—a tuning-in or making-space process, a gradual practice that adapts to your changing needs and abilities. This approach will create change that is much more sustainable.

Below is a basic four step cycle that should take about six weeks. I recommend you go through the cycle once, taking on manageable bite-sized challenges, and then circle back through it, layering on more strategies. Michelangelo famously said that his job as an artist was to chisel away the stone and reveal the form trapped inside. That's how I think of transformation. Like chiseling away at a stone, continue cycling back through this process, making more observa-

PART FOUR: Transitioning to Resilience: Finding Your 80/20

tions and layering on more strategies, but staying within your capabilities and reaching out for help and support when you need it. Do this until you have run out of strategies to implement.

Step 1: Press the reset button and get organized.
Refer back to the stressors from Part One and pick one or two to address.

Here are some things to work on (pick one or two that seem manageable):
- Replace toxic cookware.
- Assess your home's air quality and exposure to environmental contaminants.
- Replace your plastic containers with glass or stainless steel.
- Replace your cleaners and personal care products with non-toxic alternatives.
- Get an air purifier for your home or bedroom.
- Clean up the clutter and throw out the junk.
- Familiarize yourself with the Environmental Working Group's research on pesticides and start to incorporate it as best you can.
- Reorganize your pantry and familiarize yourself with new foods (see Appendix N).
- Focus on shifting bedtimes to a little earlier in the evening and/or improving sleep quality.
- Start to read food labels with an eye for the additives.
- Seek out alternative recipes and products.
- Begin reducing sugar and change your sugars to those on the low glycemic list.

Again, do as many of these as make sense for you at this time. As you cycle back, you will layer on more of these strategies once room has been made for them.

Step 2: Assess
Go back to that list you made envisioning your family's health. Work through the appendices and various checklists in this book and try to determine what factors if any, are the most likely to be contributing to road blocks. Number these in what you think is their order of importance and then start with number one. Leave the rest for the next times you pass through this cycle.

Here are some things you might want to think about:
- Do you suspect any nutrient deficiencies? See Appendix K.
- Is digestion a major issue for your child? See Appendix M and pages 111–112.
- Is unstable blood sugar triggering symptoms? See pages 91–92.
- If you have a picky eater, which of the strategies from that section does it make sense to start with? See pages 144–152.
- Do you think allergies or food sensitivities are an issue? Start a modified or full elimination diet to determine food sensitivities or get testing done. See Appendix G.

Try to get as clear a picture in your mind as you can about what is influencing your child's health. This will give you a starting point and a clear path forward.

Step 3: Implement
Add in one or more strategies from each of the core principles (see page 134–135 for a summary). Trust your gut and focus on what resonates with you. Go with what makes sense to start with based on your observations from step 2 and your health goals, and tuck the other stuff away for the next pass through the cycle of transformation.

PART FOUR: Transitioning to Resilience: Finding Your 80/20

Step 4: Consider environment.
Start to consider your eating patterns and language around food. Pick one or more strategies from Part Three to implement.

That's the four step cycle. It should take about six weeks (longer if you include an elimination diet).

Now that you've been through the cycle once, note any changes you've seen, referring back to that list you made of your health vision, and circle back to step 1. Pick one or two more things to implement. Keep going. Be consistent and strategic.

Here's an important note: I have seen incredible changes in health, growth, learning, and behaviour by implementing these strategies. But health does not change in an instant. Once you have made changes, stay the course for at least six months. If you still haven't achieved the level of health you are seeking by then, it's time to reach out for additional help. You've set a solid foundation but need to dig through more layers of complexity. It's time to work with someone to add in botanicals and high dose supplements, and facilitate testing and other therapies.

But first things first. Keep layering on the strategies for raising resilience until you have mastered them and they have become a part of your routine. Until you've grasped the strategies in this book, resist the need to know more and search more. That will only clutter the path and deplete your already stretched energy. You have a lot to start with, right here. Move slowly, systematically, be consistent, and have compassion for yourself.

Closing Thoughts

I have nothing but love and respect for you and your parenting journey. It's a hard, beautiful, and amazing process to accompany little people through childhood. We need strength and grounding to get through. We need faith, love, and courage as our companions.

You can do this. If you hate to cook, can't cook, or just don't have time, you can still do this. If you have a picky eater, you can still do this. If you have been eating processed cheese and instant noodles your whole life, you can still do this.

How? Baby steps.

Why? Because your kids will be healthier, happier, stronger, and you will be establishing a foundation for health which will culminate in fewer trips to the emergency room, fewer days home from school, and less worry. You will feel strong and confident in your ability to understand and coordinate your family's healthcare. Now is your window of opportunity, the time when you can take the wheel and steer the ship, knowing full well that at some point it will be out of your control and you will have to allow your child to set sail.

Alongside my writing of this book, a paradigm-shifting movement has been gaining momentum. It has motivated me in my mission to share what I know about physical resilience and help as many parents as possible maximize their use of food as a supportive tool for health. It's a movement made up of doctors, nutritionists, and thousands of other health care practitioners who support prevention, health promotion, and personalized health care; practitioners who empower us each to take the lead in our own health, and learn practical lifestyle tools for preventing and reversing chronic disease.

This book has evolved out of my own journey because I, like you, see the future in our children. Like you, I know healthy food needs to be a strong part of my parenting framework, but as a new mom I was confused and struggled to implement what I knew.

My drive to use my training and understanding of how food impacts the body to support my children, along with what I know first-hand of the chaotic reality of day-to-day parenting, sent me on a long search for simple, doable food and feeding strategies that would ultimately give me a massive return on my efforts. They became the core strategies for *Raising Resilience*, and I have offered them to you here in the hope you can learn from my experience and integrate them into your own food and feeding framework.

Some of the strategies here will work for you; others will not. Remember to have compassion for yourself. You are on this journey with your children. It can be a steep learning curve for you both.

If you're just starting on you this journey, start small. Make incremental changes until your family's taste buds get used to it. Enjoy new tastes and laugh about your failures along with your kids (we had a good laugh over broccoli muffins). If you are well into this, then come over to our on-line community and share your experience. It will help us all strengthen our resolve.

Above all else, don't give up. The choices you make in your kitchen have a huge impact on your health and that of your kids. Over time this will become part of a very rewarding routine.

We all love our children and yearn to see them thrive. We want them to be smart, active, and strong, and we hope they will have good judgment, positive relationships, and confidence. Ultimately, we want them to be healthy, happy, and resilient.

I wish all of this and more for you and your family.

Here's to creating and supporting vibrant health together!

Jess Sherman

Recipes for Resilience

A few words about these recipes

These recipes pull together the three core strategies for raising resilience, so you can really make this happen for your family. They call for real food ingredients, are nutrient-dense, contain lower glycemic sweeteners and other ingredients that support digestion. They are free of refined sugar, additives, refined flours, and oils. Many are dairy-free and all are gluten-free. You can find more recipes on my website at www.JessSherman.com.

NOTE: Some of you might be on specialized diets. I work with a lot of families who are, but this particular sample of recipes was not created with those protocols in mind. Having said that, because these are real food recipes most of them can easily be adapted.

A few notes about ingredients

Thickeners: To thicken soups and stews I choose to use arrowroot, tapioca, agar, or potato starch as a thickener over corn starch. Corn starch can be irritating to the gut and is less nutritive. You can also use a good quality grass-fed gelatin, thicken with puréed pumpkin or squash, or simply leave the thickener out.

Broth: You'll notice that I incorporate a lot of broth into these recipes. I consider broth to be a foundation for real food cooking. Not only does it impart a terrific flavour, but it adds a great deal of nutrition to your meals. In most recipes meat broth, stock, fish stock, and vegetable broth are interchangeable. You'll find recipes for them in the following Staples section. Using commercial broth found in tetra packs and cans is NOT the same thing. Commercial broth contributes flavour and additives, but negligible nutrition in comparison.

Nuts: Nuts are a common allergen, and many of you likely send your kids to nut-free schools or have allergies in your family. Some of these recipes (particularly the snacks and treats) involve nuts because of their nutrient density. You can generally substitute sunflower and pumpkin seeds and coconut, if tolerated.

Eggs: Eggs are also a common allergen. If you are keeping eggs out of your diet you'll find two egg replacer recipes in the Staples section.

In addition, In Appendix N, you'll find a list of whole foods to have handy.

STAPLES

Basic Ketchup

12 oz. (2 small cans) tomato paste
¼ cup water
2 tbsp apple cider vinegar
¼ tsp mustard powder
¼ tsp cinnamon
⅛ tsp cloves
⅛ tsp allspice
½ tsp sea salt
¼ cup xylitol or maple syrup
1 tsp molasses

Combine everything in a 500 ml mason jar and mix well.

Makes two cups.

TIP! For a ketchup seasoning shortcut, blend together 2 tsp each mustard powder and cinnamon, and 1 tsp each cloves and allspice. Keep this spice blend on hand and use 1 tsp spice blend for each batch of ketchup, adding together with all the other ingredients (tomato paste, water, apple cider vinegar, sea salt, xylitol or maple syrup, and molasses).

Mayonnaise

3 egg yolks (they must be at room temperature when you start)
1 tsp mustard
1½ tbsp apple cider vinegar
½ to 1 cup virgin olive oil
½ tsp sea salt

Put everything except the oil in a food processor or blender. Pulse to combine. With the machine running, add the oil in a very slow drizzle until it is all added and mixture is thick.

Cover tightly and keep in the fridge. Note that egg replacers do not work for this recipe.

Chicken Broth

Cut a whole chicken into about 8 pieces.
Place in a large pot and add enough filtered water to cover.
Bring to a low simmer and cook until chicken is done (2 to 4 hours).
Take out the chicken and debone it. Set aside the chicken to use in dishes such as curry or fajitas.
Strain the broth and use it as a base for stew, gravy, soup, etc.
Return the bones to the pot; add new water and make stock.
(See Chicken Bone Stock recipe below.)

Chicken Bone Stock

To a large stock pot, add:

All the bones from a whole, large chicken (See Chicken Broth recipe above)

2 tbsp cider vinegar

1 onion, quartered

2 large carrots, chopped into large chunks (optional)

1 tsp peppercorns (optional)

1 tsp whole cloves (optional)

Water to cover

Break the carcass into pieces to expose as much of the bone marrow as possible.

Add enough water to cover.

Add other ingredients and bring to a very low simmer. Reduce heat and simmer 12 to 24 hours.

As an option for added nutrients, add 1 bunch of parsley and 1 stick of wakame seaweed about 10 minutes before the stock is done.

Strain the broth and discard the bones and vegetables. You can either let it cool and skim off the fat that rises to the top, or you can leave the fat in (though it will be a bit greasy).

TIP! Using the meat yields a broth that is milder in flavour and higher in amino acids, while using the bones creates a broth that is more mineral-dense and higher in histamine. People with allergies, illness, or digestive upset tend to do better with the broth because it is easier to digest, however, if these are not an issue in your family, broth and stock can be used interchangeably.

Vegetable Stock

In a large pot combine:

2 potatoes, skin on, chopped into large chunks
2 carrots, chopped into large chunks
2 celery stalks, chopped into large chunks (celery leaves are good too)
Any vegetable trimmings you have (e.g. chard, kale, or broccoli stalks)
A handful of parsley
2 to 3 cloves garlic (optional)
Water to cover (about 8 cups)

Cover, bring to a boil, then simmer about 20 minutes. Strain.

TIP! Any vegetables or scraps can be used to make a mineral-rich vegetable stock. If you have a favourite bouillon, take a look at the ingredients and try using those (minus the additives, of course!)

Corn-Free Baking Powder

2 tbsp baking soda
4 tbsp arrowroot powder
4 tbsp cream of tartar

Mix well and store in a tightly closed jar. Keeps for three months.

Use 1½ times what is called for in traditional baking powder recipes. (If a recipe calls for 1 tsp baking powder, use 1½ tsp of this substitute.)

Egg Replacers

Recipe #1:
  Mix together:
  1¼ cups arrowroot flour or tapioca flour
  ¼ cup corn-free baking powder
  ½ tbsp guar gum or xanthan gum

Keep this handy, stored in a jar.

When ready to use, combine 1½ tsp of the powder with 3 tbsp water and whisk well. This equals 1 egg. Scale up as needed.

Recipe #2:
  Combine 1 tbsp ground chia seeds or flax seeds with ¼ cup water. Mix well and let it sit in the fridge until a gel forms (about 15 minutes). This equals 1 egg. Scale up as needed.

Fortified Salt

Mix ground pink Himalayan rock salt with kelp flakes in a ratio of 1:1. Store in a jar for easy use and sprinkle on as a salty seasoning for flavour and extra minerals. Use this mixture anywhere salt is called for in these recipes.

BREAKFASTS

Basic Breakfast Smoothie

¼ cup full fat coconut milk
¼ cup kefir, if tolerated (otherwise water or nut/seed milk of your choice)
1 tbsp ground flax seeds
1 tbsp hemp seeds
½ cup chopped green vegetables (spinach, chard, kale)
1 cup frozen cherries

1 small (slightly green) banana
1 serving good quality protein powder
1–2 small raw Jerusalem artichokes or 1 tbsp raw potato starch
2 to 3 drops of stevia, if desired

Place all ingredients in a high-powered blender, and blend until smooth.

Pumpkin Power French Toast

3 eggs
¼ cup full fat coconut milk
¼ cup mashed pumpkin
Dash of cinnamon
3 to 4 slices of whole grain or gluten-free bread
1 tbsp coconut oil

Beat the eggs; add the coconut milk, mashed pumpkin, and cinnamon. Dip the bread slices in the mixture to coat both sides. Fry on medium heat in coconut oil.

Rice/Millet Pudding

2 cups cooked rice or millet
1½ cups almond milk
1 cup full fat coconut milk
¼ cup maple syrup or xylitol
5 eggs, beaten
1 tbsp vanilla
1 tsp cinnamon
1 tsp nutmeg
½ cup raisins

Combine all ingredients. Pour into lightly greased baking dish. Dust with cinnamon. Bake at 375°F approximately 45 minutes, until set.

Raising Resilience

TIP! If you are having rice or millet with your dinner, make a little extra. Bake this pudding in the evening to make a great quick breakfast.

Oven Oatmeal/Quinoa

Soak overnight: 1 cup oats or quinoa in warm water, plus 1 tbsp lemon juice or yogurt.

In the morning: Drain and rinse.

Note: It will take less time to cook and be more digestible if you soak the oats, but if you forget, don't worry about it—just cook as directed.

In a pot, warm:

3 cups milk of any type, or water (or combination)
1 cup chopped apples or other fruit (dried apricots, dates, figs, etc.)
¼ cup raisins
¼ tsp nutmeg
½ tsp cinnamon

Warm until very hot, but not yet boiling
Add drained grains.
Transfer to oven-safe dish, cover and bake at 375°F for 15 to 30 minutes, while you get ready for your day.

Before serving, add:
¼ to ½ cup sunflower seeds
¼ to ½ cup hemp seeds
¼ cup ground flax or chia seeds
½ cup coconut milk
Protein powder (optional)

Recipes for Resilience

Quick and Easy Pumpkin Custard

5 eggs, slightly beaten
3 cups full fat coconut milk (or combination of milks)
1 cup puréed pumpkin
¼ cup maple syrup
¼ tsp ground cloves
⅛ tsp salt
½ tsp ground ginger
¼ tsp ground nutmeg
1 tsp cinnamon
1 tsp pure vanilla extract

Mix all ingredients in a blender. Transfer to a baking dish. Bake at 400°F for approximately 40 minutes until it's bubbling and slightly brown around the edges, and is set.

TIP! Make this the night before for a quick breakfast.

Protein-Packed Gluten-Free Pancakes

Into a high-powered blender, add the following:
1 medium plantain, peeled and broken into pieces
3 medium Jerusalem artichokes, washed and chopped; no need to peel
2 cups unsweetened almond milk (or milk of your choice)
2 eggs or egg substitute
½ cup pressed dry cottage cheese (optional, for added protein)

Blend until smooth.

Add the following to the blender:
1 cup sorghum flour
1 cup buckwheat flour
¼ cup tapioca flour
¼ cup ground flax seeds
1 tsp baking soda

Blend until smooth.

Add more milk if necessary to thin, or more buckwheat flour if needed to thicken.

Fry in coconut oil over medium heat. Top with yogurt and apple sauce.

SOUPS/SALADS

Curried Squash-Lentil Soup

2 tbsp red palm oil
1 onion, chopped
1 tbsp ground cumin
1 tbsp garam masala
2 tsp ground coriander
1 tsp salt
5 to 6 cups butternut squash, peeled, seeded, and chopped (one large squash)
2 medium sweet potatoes, peeled and cubed
6 cups homemade broth of any kind
4 to 5 dried apricots, chopped
1 cup green lentils
2-inch piece of kombu seaweed (for added minerals and better digestion)
1 cup apple sauce (or 2 apples, peeled and chopped)
1 can coconut milk
¼ cup lemon juice

In a large soup pot, sauté the onions in the oil until the onions are soft and translucent.

Add to the onions, all spices, salt, squash, sweet potato, apples (if using apple sauce, add it at the end instead), apricots, kombu, lentils, and broth.

Bring to a boil, then lower the heat and simmer for 40 to 45 minutes, until the ingredients are soft and tender.
Remove kombu. Add the coconut milk and lemon juice. Add apple sauce, if using.
Purée in a blender.

Root Vegetable Soup
1 tbsp coconut oil
1 onion, diced
1 clove garlic, diced
½ celeriac, peeled and chopped
½ butternut squash, peeled, seeded, and chopped
½ large sweet potato, peeled and chopped
½ head cauliflower, chopped
2 cups homemade broth, any kind
1 cup cooked navy beans
½ cup coconut milk
Salt and pepper to taste
Sauté the onion and garlic in the coconut oil.
Add everything else and simmer about 30 minutes, until vegetables are soft.
Blend until smooth.

Fortified Pesto-Arame Salad
Soak about a cup full of arame seaweed in warm water, about 10 minutes, until softened. Drain and set aside.
In a blender, mix together the following to make a pesto sauce:
1 cup dried basil
1 cup dried parsley
¼ cup walnuts
¼ cup sunflower seeds
¼ cup grated Parmesan cheese or nutritional yeast (for a dairy-free version)

Raising Resilience

1 to 2 cloves garlic or garlic tops
¼ cup flax oil
¼ cup olive oil
½ tsp fortified salt (see recipe in Staples section above)

Cook angel hair rice noodles or Soba noodles according to directions and toss with the arame and pesto.

A few optional additions:
Halved cherry tomatoes
¼ cup pine nuts
Leftover chicken
Canned salmon or sardines
Raw carrot or sweet potato noodles (use a julienne peeler or spiral cutter to shave a raw carrot or sweet potato into noodles)

Cameron's Salad

3 medium apples, peeled and chopped into 1-inch squares
1 English cucumber, peeled and chopped into bite-size pieces
¼ cup raisins or dried cranberries
½ cup shredded cabbage
⅛ cup raw apple cider vinegar
¼ cup olive oil

Combine everything in a bowl and mix well.

WRAPS, DIPS & SPREADS

Veggie Pâté
In a high-powered blender, combine the following ingredients:
1 raw sweet potato, peeled and chopped
1 raw white potato, peeled and chopped
1 raw large carrot, chopped
1 onion, chopped
½ cup amaranth flour
1 cup sunflower seeds
3 tbsp olive oil
3 tbsp nutritional yeast
½ tsp fortified salt (see recipe in Staples section above)
1 tbsp lemon juice
2 tbsp tamari or coconut aminos
1 tsp kelp powder

Preheat oven to 350°F.
Blend all the ingredients until smooth. Spread mixture into a glass baking dish (pâté should be about 1½ inches thick).
Bake for 1 hour. Cool.
Use in wraps with avocado, mayonnaise, sprouts, and cucumber.

Black Bean Wraps
2 cups black beans, cooked
1 small onion, chopped
2 cloves garlic, minced
1 carrot, peeled and chopped
½ cup rolled oats
¼ cup natural almond or sunflower seed butter
¼ cup unsalted, raw pumpkin seeds
3 tbsp ground flax seed

2 tbsp olive oil
1 egg or egg substitute
1 tsp each paprika, curry powder, salt
1 tbsp dried thyme

Preheat oven to 375°F.
Place all ingredients in a food processor. Process until smooth.
Transfer to a glass dish and bake about 1 hour. Cool.
Spread in a pita or wrap with lettuce, avocado, and salsa. Roll up!

Hummus 3 Ways
Traditional Hummus:
1½ cups cooked chick-peas (you can also use cooked black beans or pinto beans)
3 to 4 tbsp lemon juice
¼ cup tahini
1 small clove garlic, peeled and chopped in quarters
½ tsp ground cumin
1 tbsp umeboshi paste (fermented plum)
3 to 4 tbsp virgin olive oil
Fortified salt to taste (see recipe in Staples section above)

Put all ingredients except olive oil and salt in a food processor, and purée until smooth. With the machine on, add the olive oil in a thin stream. Season with salt to taste.

Basic Cauliflower Hummus
4 cups steamed cauliflower
2 tbsp almond butter, tahini, or sunflower seed butter
¼ cup olive oil
1 to 2 cloves garlic

1 tbsp umeboshi paste (fermented plum)
1 tsp cumin
½ tsp salt

Cool the steamed cauliflower. Add everything to a blender, and blend until smooth.

Fermented Hummus

Thank you to my colleague Lorene Sauro for the idea of fermenting the chick-peas before making the hummus. This yields a gentler flavour than if you were to make the hummus and then ferment it.

Place about 1½ cups cooked chick-peas in a large mason jar. Cover with water, leaving at least an inch of space at the top.
Add 1 tsp sea salt, plus 2 tbsp raw apple cider vinegar.
Mix well, cover tightly and let it sit on the counter one week to ferment. Periodically, you'll want to loosen the lid to let gas escape.
Drain and rinse, and use the fermented chick-peas in the traditional hummus recipe above.

Citrus Guacamole

3 ripe avocados, peeled, pitted, and coarsely chopped
2 tbsp freshly-squeezed lemon juice
1 tbsp freshly-squeezed orange juice
1 tbsp freshly-squeezed lime juice
3 cloves garlic, finely minced
1 cup packed fresh cilantro leaves
1 tsp sea salt

Combine all ingredients in a blender or food processor and pulse until smooth.
Makes 2 cups.

MAIN MEALS

Lazy Cabbage Rolls

1 lb. ground beef (or mix ½ lb. ground beef with ½ lb. ground heart and
½ cup chicken liver for added nutrition)
1 large onion, chopped
3 cloves garlic, minced
2 cups stewed tomatoes
2 cups water or broth
½ cup quinoa or brown rice
½ cup grated carrot
½ cup grated zucchini
1 tsp salt
1 tsp basil
1 tsp thyme
2 tsp oregano
½ head cabbage, shredded

In a large deep dish frying pan, sauté the onion, garlic, meat, and herbs until meat is browned.
Add all other ingredients, cover, and cook on stove top until grain is done, about 15 to 45 minutes, depending on which type of grain you use.

Quick & Easy Fish Patties

1 can wild salmon
2 cans wild sardines (in water, not oil)
½ cooked sweet potato or Jerusalem artichoke
1 egg or egg replacer
1 tbsp Dijon mustard
¼ cup almond flour

¼ cup coconut flour
⅛ cup ground flax meal
¼ cup red palm oil for frying

Place everything except the oil in a bowl. Mash the fish well and make sure all ingredients are well mixed together.
Form the batter into balls (makes about 9).
Melt the oil in a skillet and when very hot, press the balls into patties on the oil.
Cook 1 to 2 minutes on each side until golden brown.

Quick Chicken Curry

2 lb. boneless, skinless chicken thighs
1 400 ml can full fat coconut milk
1 cup homemade chicken broth
1 small tomato, chopped
2 carrots, washed and chopped (leave peel)
½ head cauliflower, chopped
1 sweet potato, peeled and chopped or 2 cups chopped butternut squash
2 cups shredded greens (spinach, kale, chard, etc.)
2 tbsp curry powder
Salt and pepper to taste

Put everything in a crock pot or soup pot. Simmer on stove top for about 1 hour, or cook in crock pot on low for 7 hours, or high for 4 hours.

Mac and Cheese (dairy-free option)

½ cup pine nuts
½ cup water or homemade broth
½ head of cauliflower, steamed

2 tbsp raw potato starch
¼ cup nutritional yeast
¼ cup shredded parmesan cheese (optional – see note below)
3 tbsp ground flax seed
1 clove garlic, chopped into quarters
½ small onion, chopped
1 tsp fortified salt
2 tsp dried basil or ¼ cup fortified pesto (see Fortified Pesto-Arame Salad)
Macaroni of your choice (quinoa, rice, wheat, etc.)

Preheat oven to 350°F.
Prepare the macaroni according to package directions.
Steam the cauliflower.
Add all the ingredients except the noodles in a blender. Blend on high until smooth.
Combine the cooked macaroni with the sauce in an oven-proof casserole dish. Bake about 20 minutes.

TIP! You can make this dairy-free by leaving out the cheese and using a bit more nutritional yeast. You can also leave out the nutritional yeast and add more cheese if desired. You can also sprinkle cheese or ground cashews on top before baking, if tolerated.

SNACKS/TREATS

Coconut-Chia Mango Pudding
2 cups whole milk or milk alternative
5 tbsp whole chia seeds + 3 tbsp ground chia seeds
1 to 2 tsp vanilla extract (or to taste)
1 to 2 tbsp maple syrup or xylitol (or to taste)
1 to 2 cups chopped mango or other fruit (fresh or frozen)

Place the milk in a bowl.

Add the chia seeds, vanilla, and sweetener, and stir to combine well. Add the fruit.

Cover and put in the fridge for 1 hour. Take it out and stir well again. Chill for another hour or two until set.

Gluten-Free Muffins

1 ripe banana, mashed
½ cup unsweetened apple sauce
⅔ cup fruit juice (pineapple, apricot, or pear work well)
⅓ cup melted coconut oil
1 tsp ginger root powder (optional)
1 tsp lemon juice (optional)
1 cup amaranth flour
½ cup buckwheat flour
1 tsp baking powder
1 tsp baking soda
½ tsp sea salt
½ cup hemp seeds, chia seeds, flax seeds, or black sesame seeds (or a combination)
1 cup coarsely chopped walnuts (optional)

Preheat oven to 350°F.

Combine mashed banana, apple sauce, fruit juice, oil, ginger, and lemon juice. In another bowl, combine flours, baking soda, baking powder, salt, and seeds.

Add the wet mixture to the dry and mix just until blended. Add walnuts.

Fill muffin tins and bake for 20 to 25 minutes. Cool before eating. Makes 9 to 12 small muffins.

Raising Resilience

Homemade Jello

½ cup cold water
2 tbsp good quality gelatin powder
½ cup hot water
3 cups natural unsweetened fruit juice

Pour the cold water into a large glass dish and add the gelatin. Stir until well mixed.
Add the hot water and stir to mix.
Add the juice and mix well.
Cover and put in the refrigerator for at least 2 hours to set.
You can add chunks of fruit as an option.

TIP! You can make this into a basic vanilla pudding by using milk or milk substitute instead of juice and water. Use the same method but dissolve 3 tbsp coconut sugar into the hot milk, and add 1 tsp vanilla extract to the pudding before you leave it to set.

Grain-Free Banana Date Muffins

2 cups ground nuts of any kind
2 tsp baking soda
1 tsp sea salt
1 tbsp cinnamon
1 cup dates, pitted (9–10)
2 ripe plantains (or 3 bananas)
3 eggs
1 tsp apple cider vinegar (or lemon juice)
¼ cup coconut oil, melted
1½ cups mixed shredded carrots and sweet potato
¾ cup walnuts (or nuts of choice), finely chopped (optional)
9 to 12 muffin paper liners

Preheat oven to 350°F.
Grind the nuts in a food processor.
In a bowl, combine the ground nuts, baking soda, salt, and cinnamon.
In a food processor, combine dates, plantains (or bananas), eggs, vinegar, and coconut oil.
Add the wet mixture to the dry mixture and combine thoroughly.
Fold in the shredded carrots, sweet potato, and nuts.
Spoon mixture into greased or paper lined muffin tins.
Bake for 25 minutes.
Cool before eating.

Black Bean Brownies

15 oz. cooked black beans
½ cup pure cocoa powder
1 tsp instant decaf coffee
3 eggs or egg replacer
2 tbsp amaranth flour
1 tbsp sorghum flour
¾ cup maple syrup
1 tbsp melted butter or coconut oil
1 tsp vanilla extract

Preheat oven to 350°F.
Combine the beans, cocoa, coffee, eggs, and flours and process in a food processor until smooth.
Add in the maple syrup, oil and vanilla and process another minute or so.
Pour into a greased pan and bake for about 20 minutes.
Turn down the oven to 300°F and bake another 5 to 10 minutes.
Cool, transfer to the fridge and chill about 3 hours before cutting.

Raising Resilience

Golden Tea (Turmeric Tea)

Make a Turmeric tea or paste:

If using powdered spices:

Combine ¼ cup turmeric powder, ⅛ cup ginger root powder, 1 tsp ground black pepper with ½ cup water. Heat in a saucepan for about 3 to 5 minutes until a paste forms. Transfer to a jar and store in the fridge until ready to use.

If using roots:

Combine 3 to 4 chopped turmeric tubers, 1-inch knob chopped ginger root, 1 to 2 tsp black peppercorns, with 2 cups water. Simmer 10 minutes on low to make a strong tea. Strain. Store this in the fridge until ready to use.

To make the tea, combine:

½ cup coconut milk or almond milk (if you use almond milk, add a bit of coconut oil—the fat helps the absorption of the curcumin), ½ cup coconut water (or you can leave this out and use 1 cup milk instead), approximately ½ tsp turmeric paste or ½ cup turmeric tea (you can do this to taste). A pinch cinnamon (optional).

Heat and add honey to taste.

Digestive Tea

To get the digestive juices flowing and relieve digestive upset.

1-inch ginger root, chopped
3 to 4 medium turmeric roots, chopped
1 tbsp coriander seeds
1 tbsp fennel seeds
1 small cinnamon stick
½ cup dried lemon balm leaves
½ cup dried peppermint leaves

In a small pot, combine the first five ingredients with 2½ cups water. Cover and bring to a boil. Simmer about 15 to 20 minutes. Remove the pot from heat, add the leaves, cover, and let steep another 10 minutes. Strain the tea. Add ½ cup coconut milk. Sweeten with raw honey to taste and dilute with water or more milk if it's too strong tasting. Store this tea in the fridge and reheat as needed.

FABULOUS FERMENTS

NOTE: Never use chlorinated tap water; use only filtered or spring water. Chlorine will kill the bacteria and fermentation will not occur (honey and iodized salt also weaken bacteria).

Basic Brine

You can use this basic brine for all vegetable ferments except sauerkraut.

Mix together about 3 tbsp salt and 4 cups water. Your brine should taste like sea water.

Fermented Carrot Sticks

Pack a 500 ml wide-mouth mason jar with peeled carrot sticks (about 6 medium carrots). Cut them short enough so that you have about 1-inch of space at the top.

Add 1 tbsp of fresh dill (or 1 tsp dried), and 2 cloves peeled garlic.

Add enough basic brine to fully submerge the carrots.

Cover and let it sit at room temperature for about 3 to 7 days.

TIP! You can use this same basic process for any vegetable sticks or chunks like jicama, turnip, beets, beans, radish.

Raising Resilience

Fermented Ketchup

Make the Ketchup recipe found in the Staples recipe section, using maple syrup as your sweetener. In place of water, add homemade whey (make this by placing a strainer over a bowl and lining it with a cotton dish towel. Pour plain, good quality yogurt into the strainer and let it sit. The whey is the liquid that drips through into the bowl).

Put everything in a 500 ml mason jar. Leave about an inch at the top. Mix or shake well to combine. Cover with a lid and ferment at room temperature for about 4 to 5 days. When it has reached a flavour you like, store it in the fridge to stop the fermentation process.

Probiotic Lemonade

Juice of 5 lemons

¼ to ⅓ cup pure organic cane sugar

½ cup homemade whey (see Fermented Ketchup recipe above for directions)

5 cups (approximately) filtered water

Combine everything in a 1.5 L mason jar. Fill the jar with the filtered water. Cover and shake gently to combine. Ferment at room temperature for 2 to 5 days. Transfer to the fridge and chill before drinking.

Basic Sauerkraut

1. Remove the outer 2 to 3 leaves of a whole red or green cabbage and set aside.
2. Shred or chop the entire cabbage head into a bowl.
3. Sprinkle 2 tsp salt over.
4. Massage the cabbage until the juices release (about 5 minutes. See tip below).
5. Taste the cabbage. It should taste like sea water. Add salt as necessary.
6. You want to have about ¼ cup liquid brine in the bowl. If you don't, add some spring water and keep tasting it. Add salt as necessary to keep that sea water-like taste.
7. Pack a 1.5 L wide mouth jar with the cabbage. Pack it down as much as you can with your fist. Pour in any liquid from the bowl. Make sure the shredded cabbage is covered with liquid. Add a bit more fresh water if you need to, but leave about 2 inches at the top as gasses will accumulate.
8. Roll up the 2 to 3 cabbage leaves you've set aside and place them over the shredded cabbage so they take up the extra space and pack down the kraut. Cover with a lid, but not too tightly, so gasses can escape.
9. Let it sit on the counter for at least 5 days. Keep tasting it after that and when you like the taste transfer to cold storage to slow down the fermentation.

TIP! After shredding the cabbage, sprinkle on the salt, mix with your hands, and let it sit. The cabbage will wilt and become easier to massage.

APPENDICES

Appendix A   Important Micronutrients and Where to Find Them
Appendix B   Enzymes, Bacteria, and Fibre: The Forgotten Players
Appendix C   Non-Dairy Sources of Calcium
Appendix D   Traditional Food Preparation
Appendix E   Signs and Symptoms of Food Allergy
Appendix F   Fatty Acid Deficiency: Detecting and Correcting
Appendix G   Elimination Diet
Appendix H   Gluten or Gluten-Free?
Appendix I   Choosing Supplements
Appendix J   Phenols in Foods
Appendix K   Common Deficiency Symptoms
Appendix L   Glutamate and Additives
Appendix M   Common Signs of Gut Dysbiosis
Appendix N   Whole Foods to Have Handy

APPENDIX A

Important Micronutrients and Where to Find Them

Calcium

Calcium is essential for growing children. Our bones develop until the age of thirty, after which they start to deteriorate. If we develop strong bones when we're younger, then there will be more mass when deterioration begins and osteoporosis is less likely. Our teeth also need adequate calcium for proper formation and health.

Concern about calcium deficiency should include a look at how calcium is excreted from the body. It's not terribly difficult for your child to get enough calcium if it is being properly absorbed and not excreted in the urine.

Some things that leach calcium from the body are:
- soda
- chocolate
- refined sugar
- phosphorus (in meat, grain, soft drinks, additives)
- salt
- excess fibre
- lack of vitamin D
- excess protein
- second hand smoke
- corticosteroid medication

While it is true that milk is a source of calcium, there are a few reasons to approach cow's milk with caution.

Raising Resilience

1. Pasteurized cow's milk is the number one allergen among kids. One of two proteins, Casein and Beta Lacto globulin, usually cause the problem. Often, early sensitivities to milk go unnoticed and lead to further complications later.
2. Commercial milk has been pasteurized at very high heat. This changes the protein structures and kills off beneficial bacteria and enzymes, making milk somewhat difficult to digest and making the calcium it offers poorly absorbed by many children.
3. The homogenization process that milk undergoes requires that the milk be spun in a centrifuge to break up the fat and protein molecules. This process also makes the milk harder to digest.
4. Some kids get addicted to milk and drink too much of it. This is problematic for several reasons:
   a) It may indicate a sensitivity; we often crave what we are allergic to (see the section on allergies).
   b) It might supply too much calcium. Calcium binds to zinc and iron, preventing their absorption.
   c) Milk may fill up your child and take the place of other foods that provide a more diverse nutrient base.

Cultured milk, like plain yogurt or kefir, is much easier to digest and introduces good bacteria that helps keep the digestive flora healthy and balanced. The calcium in cultured milk is easier to absorb than the calcium found in uncultured milk.

Calcium needs fat in order to be metabolized, so avoid low-fat yogurts (they tend to have all sorts of additives and added sugar in them anyhow). Also avoid sweetened yogurts (with natural or artificial sweeteners), and yogurts with added fruit.

If you do choose to give dairy, sixteen ounces of high fat dairy a day will give a child the calcium she needs without overdoing it.

See Appendix C for a list of non-dairy foods that are high in calcium, and calcium needs for kids.

Zinc

Zinc is involved in dozens of the body's chemical processes including metabolism, cell, and tissue synthesis and the development of bones and cognitive function. It is essential for building the immune system.

Zinc is involved in the senses of taste and smell. A child who is a very picky eater, is lacking in appetite, or often insists that foods smell too strong or taste off, is often deficient in zinc.

Sources of Zinc:
The best source is oysters, followed by pumpkin seeds. The following are also good sources:
- liver
- beef
- salmon
- sunflower seeds
- molasses
- oats
- green and split peas
- eggs
- chicken
- almonds
- blackeye peas
- brown rice
- buckwheat
- pecans

Iron

Iron is essential for building of the immune system and for proper growth. Deficiencies in iron have also been linked with poor cognitive development,[114] and increased hyperactivity.[115]

Raising Resilience

There are two different types of iron: Heme iron is found in animal sources; non-heme iron is found in grains, fruits, and vegetables.

Iron metabolism is aided by vitamin C, so try to combine your iron foods with vitamin C-rich foods. Iron absorption is inhibited by too much calcium.

Sources of Iron:
None of these alone (except liver) will provide enough iron, so combine them and integrate them into dishes:
- liver
- salmon
- blackstrap molasses
- oats
- kidney beans
- blackeye peas
- Kamut
- spinach
- sunflower seeds
- beef
- raisins
- lentils
- quinoa
- black beans
- clams
- chicken
- spirulina
- eggs
- dulse (seaweed)
- apricots
- chick-peas
- black sesame seeds
- dried prunes

Vitamin A

Vitamin A is essential for proper eye, mucous membrane, neurological development, and immune function. Vitamin A is also involved in regulating growth, so deficiencies can lead to painful growth spurts.

Preformed vitamin A is only found in animal foods. The form found in fruits and vegetable is called beta-carotene. The body is able to transform beta-carotene into vitamin A.

Babies are not able to make this transformation well, so they need to be given foods with preformed vitamin A.[116] Toddlers are better converters, but they need adequate cofactors (vitamins and enzymes) in order to be able to do it.

Vitamin A is a fat-soluble vitamin, so fat is needed for its absorption.

Sources of Vitamin A and Beta-Carotene:

Vitamin A
- eggs
- liver
- whole fortified milk
- raw milk
- butter
- cod liver oil

Beta-Carotene
- sweet potatoes
- pumpkins
- carrots
- squash
- spinach
- broccoli
- tomatoes
- apricots
- parsley
- green leafy vegetables

Raising Resilience

TIP: Adding some saturated fat (butter, cream, or coconut oil) to your mashed vegetables will help the conversion of beta-carotene to vitamin A and the absorption of vitamin A.

Vitamin D

This vitamin, along with several others, is essential for the metabolism of calcium and phosphorus. Healthy bones are dependent on vitamin D. New research is showing vitamin D as a player in hundreds of chemical activities and there are vitamin D receptors all over the body.

Sources of Vitamin D:
- liver
- butter
- sardines
- vitamin D fortified milk
- raw milk
- eggs
- Swiss cheese
- sunshine (only if adequate cholesterol is present)
- cod liver oil

Magnesium

Magnesium is essential to over three hundred chemical reactions including proper bone development, proper muscle and nerve function, blood sugar management, enzyme function, protein synthesis, and metabolism of vitamin D and calcium.

Magnesium is a calming mineral, and deficiency has been linked to hyperactivity and muscle cramps.

The magnesium level of food is dependent on the magnesium level of the soil in which it is grown. Since soil is generally being depleted of this mineral, the sources I'm listing here are purely theoretical sources of magnesium. This is one of the reasons why it's important to source good quality foods as much as possible.

Sources of Magnesium:
- beans
- almonds
- oats
- molasses
- coconut
- apricots
- green leafy vegetables
- buckwheat
- seeds
- tofu
- millet
- figs
- dates

It is quite easy to supplement with magnesium. It can be purchased as a powder, liquid, or topical oil or spray.

APPENDIX B

Enzymes, Bacteria, and Fibre: The Forgotten Players

Enzymes

Enzymes can be thought of as the workers who keep the body functioning. Every single process that occurs in the body is dependent on enzymes. The body makes some, but can become deficient. Most people with allergies need extra enzymes.

Food Sources of Enzymes:
- fermented foods like kefir, sauerkraut, and miso
- sprouted seeds
- grains and beans
- vegetable juice
- fresh, crisp vegetables

Bacteria

Our digestive tract contains about 2 kg. of bacteria, and we are learning more and more about the importance of maintaining the delicate microbiome of our bodies.

Food Sources of Bacteria:
- good quality yogurt and kefir (use them to make smoothies, popsicles, mix with fruit, or use in salad dressings and baking)
- sauerkraut
- kimchi
- miso
- tempeh

- water kefir
- kombucha
- lacto-fermented vegetables

A good quality probiotic supplement can also provide important bacteria but does not offer the same diversity as food sources.

Fibre

Fibre keeps the colon clean, adds bulk to stools, and binds to metals, cholesterol, and toxins so they can be excreted. It is also fermented into important fatty acids by intestinal microbes. Fibre generally keeps the bowels and digestion functioning well.

Food Sources of Fibre:
- whole grains (sprouted grains are best)
- seeds
- nuts
- beans
- fruit
- whole grain pasta
- whole grain bread
- raw and cooked vegetables

APPENDIX C

Non-Dairy Sources of Calcium

It's best to include as many sources as you can, rather than relying on only a few.

- black sesame seeds
- white sesame seeds and tahini
- almonds and almond butter
- hazelnuts and hazelnut butter
- sunflower seeds and sunflower seed butter
- walnuts
- canned sardines (including bones)
- canned wild salmon (including bones)
- tofu (use this only occasionally)
- homemade bone broths
- blackstrap molasses
- wakame (add this sea vegetable to soups and broths)
- swiss chard
- kale
- parsley
- green beans
- asparagus
- peas
- broccoli
- carrots
- avocados
- spinach
- navy beans
- pinto beans
- chick-peas

- kidney beans
- wild rice
- brown rice
- kelp (add kelp powder to baking)

How Much is Enough?
Recommended Daily Amount (RDA) for Calcium:
Ages 1 to 3:   500 mg. per day
Ages 4 to 8:   700 to 800 mg. per day
Ages 9 to 18:   1300 mg. per day

Some Examples:
½ cup white sesame seeds   1,100 mg.
1 cup almonds   600 mg.
1 cup sunflower seeds   260 mg.
1 cup walnuts   216 mg.
2 oz. sesame butter   842 mg.
2 oz. almond butter   225 mg.
½ cup swiss chard   51 mg.
½ cup kale   47 mg.
½ cup green beans   29 mg.
½ cup peas   22 mg.
½ cup broccoli   21 mg.
carrot (1 medium)   19 mg.
avocado (1 medium)   19 mg.
1 cup tofu   258 mg.
1 cup chick-peas   80 mg.
1 cup kidney beans   50 mg.
1 cup wild rice   30 mg.
1 cup brown rice   23 mg.
3 oz. sardines   375 mg.
3 oz. salmon   203 mg.
1 tbsp blackstrap molasses 137 mg.
1 cup whole milk   276 mg.

APPENDIX D

Traditional Food Preparation

Anthropological studies tell us that cultures around the world have practiced and passed down traditional methods of food preparation that make certain foods more digestible. In some cases these methods actually increase nutrient density as well. Western cultures have lost much of this traditional wisdom, instead favouring quick cooking methods and long shelf lives. Our health is suffering because of it. There's much more information on this topic than we can fully share here, but it's so important that it needs to be mentioned. Here are the basics:

1. **Whole Grains.** To improve digestibility of whole grains, place them in a large bowl, cover with warm water plus 1 tbsp of yogurt, lemon juice, or apple cider vinegar. Keep it in a warm place overnight. After soaking, rinse and cook the grains in new water.
2. **Nuts.** To improve digestibility, soak nuts in salt water brine overnight, and then dry them in the oven or dehydrator before eating (use about 1 tbsp of sea salt per 4 cups of nuts, cover with filtered water). TIP: For almonds, most of the anti-nutrients are in the skin. Buying slivered or blanched almonds can be a quick alternative to soaking.
3. **Meat.** Slow cooking meat preserves the delicate essential fatty acids. Don't overcook your meat (particularly if it is grass-finished).
4. **Heat.** Cook over medium-low heat when you can, and avoid overcooking foods. Deep fry only in moderation, if at all.
5. **Fermentation.** This traditional method of preserving food uses Lactobacillus bacteria, and sometimes yeast and salt, to create an environment in which pathogenic bacteria cannot grow. Lacto-

fermented foods contain no vinegar, pectin, gelatin, additives, or baker's yeast, and are very good sources of probiotic bacteria, enzymes, and vitamins. Every traditional society includes some sort of fermented food. Some examples: natto, kimchi, kefir, kombucha, pickles, sauerkraut, miso.

6. **Sourdough**. A proper sourdough bread contains grain flour which has been fermented using wild yeast that lives naturally in the environment. The sourdough process creates a bread that is easier to digest and that has less of an impact on blood sugar than a loaf made with baker's yeast. A proper sourdough bread will not contain "yeast" in the ingredients.

APPENDIX E

Signs and Symptoms of Allergies

The most common food allergies are to the following:
- wheat
- dairy
- corn
- soy
- eggs (especially whites)
- refined sugar
- beef
- caffeine
- chemicals (additives, pesticides, preservatives, dyes)
- chocolate
- citrus fruit (orange, grapefruit, lemon, lime)
- peanuts
- tree nuts
- shellfish
- strawberries
- tomatoes
- yeast

Some of the most common symptoms among babies are:

- gas
- fussiness
- constipation
- diarrhea
- eczema
- mucousy cough
- perpetually runny nose

Appendices

- bright red cheeks
- diaper rash
- thrush
- sleeplessness

Some additional common symptoms among older children are:

- behaviour and hyperactivity issues
- depression
- headaches
- sleepiness
- dark circles under the eyes

Some more medically recognized symptoms of allergies are:

- headaches
- depression
- fatigue
- moodiness
- hyperactivity
- joint pain
- irregular heart beat
- asthma
- runny nose
- abdominal pain
- excessive gas
- acne
- eczema
- itching
- muscle pain
- bed-wetting
- tinnitus
- sinusitis

Note: Symptoms of a food allergy may show up to four days after exposure.

APPENDIX F

Fatty Acid Deficiency: Detecting and Correcting

If you answer YES to three or more of the following questions, you might try making diet changes to correct an omega 3 deficiency.

Does your child exhibit any of these symptoms?

Symptom	Yes	No
Dry skin		
Brittle nails		
Bumps on the back of the upper arm		
Excessive thirst		
Lowered immunity (gets sick often and typically takes more than three days to kick it)		
Dandruff		
Trouble learning		
Irritability		
Fatigue		
Frequent infections (simple colds typically develop into more serious infections)		
Hyperactivity		
Poor wound healing		
Allergies		
Eczema		
Depression		
Anxiety		
Aggression		
Constipation		
Greasy stools		

What to Do

Correcting symptoms of fatty acid deficiency can be approached from different perspectives: reduce the omega 6s, increase the omega 3s, and/or improve the quality. I generally recommend doing all of these.

Step 1: Examine and Shift the Diet
First, look to see what your child is currently eating. Conventional meat and eggs, farmed fish, nuts and seeds, and seed and vegetable oil are very high in omega 6. Algae, wild fish, meat raised on pasture and omega 3 fortified eggs are higher in omega 3s.

How to get a more balanced ratio of 3:6:
Incorporate a variety of the following;
- seeds (hemp seeds, sesame seeds, pumpkin seeds, flax seeds and flax oil, chia seeds)
- omega 3 eggs or eggs from pasture raised chicken
- sardines
- green leafy vegetables
- nuts and nut oils (walnuts, almonds, hazelnuts, pecans)
- grass-fed meat
- seaweed (arame, kombu, nori, wakame)
- wild salmon

Avoid:
- vegetable oils (corn, soy, canola)
- conventional eggs
- conventional meat
- processed food

Step 2: Supplementation
If you want to supplement because you don't think your child's diet is cutting it, here are a few tips:
   a) Make sure to get a good quality fish oil supplement that has been tested and purified for toxins such as heavy metals and pesticide residue. Give your school-aged child about 1,000 mg. or 1 g. total fish oil, less for younger kids. For some children, too much fish oil is overstimulating, which can worsen hyperactivity and anxiety. If you see symptoms increase in your child after starting fish oil, stop.

b) Cod liver oil is another great source of EFAs but the levels are typically lower than what you'll get in a fish oil. Cod liver oil is a good source of vitamins A and D, and is a great supplement for kids, but it is NOT the same as fish oil.
c) If you are a vegetarian, you can find some EFA supplements made from algae. These tend to be much less potent than what you'll find in a fish oil, so you'll have to adjust the dosage.
d) Flax seed oil does not offer DHA and EPA, the omega 3 fatty acids critical for brain and eye development. Flax oil provides ALA, a type of omega 3 which needs to be converted in the body. Many factors get in the way of this conversion including:
  - excessive stress hormones
  - chronic infections
  - certain pharmaceutical drugs
  - tobacco smoke
  - heavy metals
  - pesticides
  - trans fatty acids
  - too much omega 6 in the diet

Fish oil offers preformed DHA and EPA.

Step 3: Maximize Nutrient Density

Simply giving a supplement is not the end of the story when it comes to EFA deficiency. In order for the body to be able to use that supplement you have to make sure that all the cofactors are in place to metabolize it. A cofactor is something needed for the proper metabolism of something else. There are several vitamins, minerals, fats, and enzymes needed in order for the body to use an omega 3 supplement. So the supplement is only one part of a bigger picture that includes an overall, nutrient-dense diet. Refer back to Core Principle #1 and Appendix A.

What about EFA-fortified foods?

1. I'm doubtful that the quality of these fats is very high. And quality is important when it comes to polyunsaturated fat (they are very unstable and can de-nature quickly).
2. The amount you get is minimal and unlikely to really make much difference, even though you pay a much higher price.
3. Many of these foods have other nasty ingredients like sugar, colouring, trans fat, refined flour, and other things. Adding a bit of fatty acid is a marketing gimmick that makes you think you're buying a product that is healthier than it likely actually is.

Appendix G

How to Do an Elimination Diet

An elimination diet consists of two stages – the Elimination Phase and the Reintroduction Phase. There are two versions of the Elimination Phase explained here: a simplified version, which is simpler but less comprehensive, and a full version which is more complete but can be difficult to manage. Do whichever you think you will be more successful at implementing.

Getting Ready

The best time to do an elimination diet is when you have a stretch of at least eight weeks during which you have complete control over your diet. Will you be traveling? Are there special holidays? Consider your timing carefully.

You may need to work up to the test diet, depending on your starting point. Some people wean themselves onto it over a period of a few weeks. It is far more effective and easier if your entire family follows the diet together.

The Elimination Phase: Simplified Version

For a minimum of ten days, eliminate wheat, dairy, eggs, soy, sugar, and corn, along with any foods you suspect or know from testing might be causing a reaction. If you can continue for twenty-one days, that is even better. If you can't do all of these common allergens, do as many as you can. Be sure to check food labels and exclude foods and additives derived from those foods as well (like soy lecithin, maltodextrine, and milk solids).

The Elimination Phase: Full Version

This approach is much more comprehensive but trickier to do. This version requires that you remove all packaged and pre-made foods since they often contain hidden ingredients.

Eliminate the following common allergens for ten to twenty-one days:
- junk food including chips, chocolate, candies, processed foods, food additives
- all dairy including goat cheese, milk, yogurt, milk solids, ice cream, modified milk ingredients, whey, casein, lactose
- eggs
- wheat (durum, semolina, breads, pasta)
- Kamut
- spelt
- barley
- rye
- non-fermented soy (beans, milk, tofu, soybean oil, soy protein isolate, textured vegetable protein)
- corn (corn chips, corn starch, corn meal, maltodextrin – see list of additives, most of them come from corn)
- sugar including glucose, fructose, corn syrup, sucrose, artificial sweeteners
- hydrogenated or partially hydrogenated oil
- margarine
- deep fried foods
- coffee
- alcohol
- mushrooms
- yeast (cakes, all bread including sourdough, yeast extract)
- peanuts
- vinegar (small amounts of apple cider vinegar is okay)
- citrus (orange, grapefruit, lime – small amounts of lemon is okay)
- processed meats

OH MY GOODNESS! WHAT CAN I EAT??? FOODS TO KEEP IN STOCK

Grains	Quick Breakfasts (check labels carefully!)	Flours	Pasta
buckwheat/kasha gluten-free steel cut oats rice (basmati, wild, brown, white) millet amaranth quinoa	puffed rice puffed millet quick rolled oats cream of rice any hot or cold cereal that does not contain gluten or corn	buckwheat flour amaranth flour chick-pea flour tapioca flour rice flour gluten-free flour mix (check for corn) almond flour coconut flour sorghum flour	rice noodles Japanese potato noodles (Saifun) quinoa noodles soba noodles kelp noodles (be sure to check ingredients for corn)

Baking Needs	Oils	Seasonings	Beans
aluminium and corn starch-free baking powder arrowroot powder agar-agar egg replacer (no corn starch) pure vanilla extract	cold pressed olive oil flax oil coconut oil organic safflower oil in small amounts red palm oil	all herbs and spices coconut aminos pure fish sauce Dijon mustard apple cider vinegar gomasio small amounts of red star nutritional yeast garlic ginger dulse vanilla	chick-peas black beans split peas kidney beans lentils adzuki beans mung beans blackeye peas

Vegetables/Fruits	Dried Fruits	Nuts and Seeds and their butters (no added oil or sugar, not roasted)	Meat, Poultry, and Fish
all vegetables are okay, fresh or frozen all fruit is okay except citrus sea vegetable	raisins apricots apples dates figs sun dried tomatoes cranberries coconut	almonds Brazil nuts cashews hazelnuts pecans pistachios pumpkin seeds walnuts sesame seeds (black and white) sunflower seeds flax seeds hemp seeds chia seeds tahini	all animal meats and shellfish are okay

Cans/Jars (check labels carefully!)	Beverages	Sweeteners (small amounts only)
organic tomato sauce organic tomato paste olives artichoke hearts salsa unsweetened apple butter unsweetened apple sauce canned sardines and salmon canned coconut milk (check ingredients) puréed pumpkin	small amounts of fruit juice is okay, no citrus juice rice milk (check labels) almond milk (check labels) lots of water herbal teas vegetable juices be sure all beverages are unsweetened	maple syrup black strap molasses honey brown rice syrup apple butter stevia xylitol coconut nectar

Menu Ideas (See the Recipes for Resilience section and my website, www.JessSherman.com)

Breakfast ideas: Vegetable juice, dairy-free smoothie, fresh fruit, nut butter on rice crackers, cream of millet, cream of rice, gluten-free oatmeal, buckwheat pancakes with almond butter and molasses, cold gluten-free cereal with almond milk or coconut yogurt

Lunch ideas: gluten-free flat bread with hummus, avocado, black bean spread, sprouts, nut butter (not peanut), fresh fruit, rice crackers, homemade bars, gluten-free muffins, homemade soups

Dinner ideas: chicken stir fry with rice, beef, and/or vegetable stews (avoid commercial broths), fish with sweet potato

Snack ideas: sesame bar, nuts, veggies and dip, zucchini carrot muffin, no-bake cookie balls, smoothies, sweet potato chips

The Reintroduction Phase

After ten to twenty-one days on either of the Elimination Phase diets, you can start re-introducing foods one at a time, every four days. Use the chart below to keep track of symptoms. Be careful, though, that you are adding one food at a time. Bread, for example, might contain wheat, soy, and corn. Instead, perhaps try a cream of wheat cereal made with coconut milk.

When you are testing a certain food, have your child eat it at least three times a day for three or four days.

It doesn't really matter what order you introduce foods. The following order is recommended for ease, but is not critical:

1. sugar (sugar on its own—like sugar-sweetened lemonade)
2. eggs
3. gluten grains (rye, barley, wheat, Kamut, spelt—one at a time. crispbreads like Ryvita are usually good choices)
4. yeast (try bread—but check the ingredients for dairy, corn and soy!)
5. dairy (butter, then yogurt, then cheese, then milk)
6. corn
7. soy
8. vinegar
9. mushrooms
10. citrus
11. peanuts
12. alcohol
13. coffee
14. chocolate

Some Symptoms to Watch For

Neurological: headaches, fatigue, hyperactivity, lethargy, moodiness, anxiety, impatience, frustration, sleeplessness, defiance, out-of-control behaviour, brain fog, poor memory, aggression

Digestive/gastro/urinary: bloating, constipation, diarrhea, gas, bed-wetting

Skin: rashes, itch, swelling

Other: achy bones or muscles, stiffness, rapid heartbeat, excessive thirst, congestion, nausea

It's extremely important to go one at a time, and honestly record signs and symptoms. Record any and all feelings, even if you think they are unrelated.

If no symptoms are seen or felt, add that food back in to the diet. If a symptom is seen or felt note it down and keep that food out for the rest of the reintroduction phase.

Raising Resilience

QUICK NOTE:
Symptoms can appear when you take the foods out and/or when you reintroduce the foods.

Food Reintroduction Chart

Ingredient (e.g. wheat, rice)	Date	Food (e.g. cracker, rice cake)	Symptom(s)	No. of days after eaten

Appendix H

Gluten or Gluten-Free?

Gluten is a family of proteins found in grains. Wheat, rye, barley, spelt, and Kamut have variations of this protein that are irritating to many people, and so are termed gluten-grains. Some people are only sensitive to the type of gluten found in wheat; others might react to them all.

In fact, there are many types of gluten. Many of them have not yet been studied. If you want to avoid gluten completely, you'll likely need a diet that is totally grain-free. But for many people, certain types of gluten are tolerable whereas others are not.

Oats can be tolerated by many people with gluten sensitivities. However, oats are often cross-contaminated with gluten if they have been processed in a facility that also processes gluten-grains. This is why you sometimes see gluten-free oats. Spelt has a very delicate form of gluten that is also easier to digest, so it is tolerated by some.

The problem with gluten stems from the fact that humans lack the enzymes needed to fully break it down into single amino acids. In those of us with very healthy gut microbes, bacteria takes up the slack when these undigested proteins enter the colon.

Celiac disease is an autoimmune disease in which the immune system is triggered by gluten to attack the intestinal lining. Non-celiac gluten sensitivity, only really confirmed to exist in 2011, is a reaction to gluten that does not involve auto-antibodies. Symptoms of non-celiac gluten sensitivity can include headaches, fuzzy thinking, fatigue, bloating, constipation, diarrhea, depression, anxiety, and much more.

If you are feeling anything less than optimal, doing a six week gluten-free experiment is a good idea. It will lift a burden from the body and free up some energy for healing.

The first step of going gluten-free is to avoid wheat, rye, and barley. However, the complexity sets in when we start to realize all the ingredients that are derived from these grains. These derivatives must be avoided as well.

Sticking with whole, unprocessed foods is the best way to avoid gluten.

Also, since all grains contain some configuration of gluten, if you don't see the results you're after by taking this first step, you might need to go a step deeper and try Paleo for a while.

Appendices

Foods Containing Gluten

Most commonly reactive gluten-containing grains, flours, and starches:	Some prepared foods that likely contain gluten:	Gluten-containing additives
barley	alcohol (like beer, wine, whiskey; gluten-free beer is available)	malt syrup
bulgur	baked beans	malt extract
couscous	breading	malt flavouring
durum	chocolate bars	malt vinegar
einkorn	dry roasted nuts	modified food starch
emmer (another name for durum)	seasoned nuts	rice malt
farro	dried fruit (sometimes dusted with wheat)	vegetable starch
graham flour	deli meats	artificial colour
Kamut	gravy	caramel colour
malt (extract, flavouring, malt syrup, vinegar)	icings and frostings	maltose
oats (oat bran, oat syrup)	imitation bacon bits	maltodextrin
rye	imitation seafood	MSG
semolina	licorice	dextrin
spelt	marinades	brown rice syrup
triticale	pastas	hydrolyzed plant protein
wheat (bran, germ, starch)	processed meats	
orzo	salad dressings	
matzoh meal	sauces	
udon	canned soups	
	seitan	
	textured vegetable protein	
	sausage products	
	seasonings	
	soups, soup bases, broth, bouillon cubes	
	soy sauce (can get wheat-free)	
	stuffing	
	supplements	
	thickeners	
	flavoured teas and coffees, herbal teas	
	non-dairy beverages	
	flavoured alcoholic beverages	
	cocoa drinks like Ovaltine	
	some coffee substitutes	
	Worchestershire sauce	
	some baking powders	
	some ice creams	

Nutritional Concerns for the Gluten-Free Diet:

Common Deficiencies	Good Food Sources
Calcium (often deficient in gluten-sensitive people)	kelp, dulse, green vegetables (especially collard greens, kale, turnip greens, dandelion greens), amaranth, quinoa, buckwheat, millet, salmon, sardines, almonds, brewer's yeast, parsley, watercress, dried figs, sunflower seeds, broccoli, calcium fortified orange juice, teff
Iron (often deficient in gluten-sensitive people)	meats, clams, oysters, lentils, blackstrap molasses, chick-peas, beans (especially pinto, black, kidney), blackeye peas, green vegetables (especially Swiss chard, turnip greens, spinach, watercress, purslane), prune juice, potatoes, sesame, sunflower, peas, dried fruit (especially figs and apricots), pumpkin seed, quinoa, millet
Fibre	nuts, nut butters, vegetables, fresh and dried fruit, flax seed, chia seed, psyllium seed, seaweeds, whole grains that are allowed (see chart), especially amaranth, teff
B vitamins	torula or brewer's yeast (note that some gluten lists warn to stay away from brewer's yeast—check with the manufacturer), sunflower seeds, pine nuts, calf liver, almonds, amaranth, buckwheat
Folate	same as that listed for B vitamins as well as: leafy greens (spinach, chard, kale, beet greens), asparagus, broccoli, cabbage, blackeye peas, beans (especially kidney, mung, lima, navy), chick-peas, lentils, walnuts

Cooking Tips:

Gluten is what gives baked goods elasticity and fluffiness and helps dough to rise, so you can expect that gluten-free baked goods will not have the same texture. Here are some tips for gluten-free baking:

When baking with gluten-free flours, combine 1 tsp xanthan gum for every cup of flour (add to dry ingredients), to maintain texture and prevent crumbling.

Good nutrient-dense flours to use include almond, amaranth, bean, pea, quinoa, teff, buckwheat, and sorghum.

When using gluten-free flours, the best results come from mixing two to three of them together and being sure to include some starch (potato, arrowroot, or tapioca) in a ratio of 1 cup flour mix: ½ cup starch.

APPENDIX I

Choosing Supplements

It's important to be a cautious consumer when it comes to supplements. In general, you get what you pay for. Here are some things to look for and learn about so you can ensure you are buying the best quality.

1. Nutrient Form

Most vitamins can be added to supplements in different forms which metabolize a bit differently in the body.

Folic acid is an example. About thirty percent of us don't efficiently transform folic acid into folate, the form of this B vitamin the body can use. Taking a supplement with the Methyltetrahydrofolate or folinic acid forms that the body doesn't need to convert is usually a better choice, although it might be more expensive.

B12 is another example. Cheaper supplements often contain the form cyanocobalamin which is typically absorbed less effectively than the methylcobalamin form you'll find in higher quality supplements.

2. Purity

PCBs, dioxins, pesticides, metals, etc., are becoming an increasingly bigger problem. We are usually taking supplements to help our bodies stay healthy; we don't want our supplements to be another source of toxicity.

Look for purity statements on your supplements. Some also have been analyzed by third party groups such as Good Manufacturing Practices (GMP), United States Pharmacopea (USP), and NSF International.

3. Potency

Many supplements, particularly those for children, contain very low, sometimes insignificant, doses of nutrients. In some multivitamins, for example, certain vitamins may be left out completely. Fish oils are another supplement that is often very low in potency. Cheaper brands and broad spectrum supplements, like multivitamins, generally contain lower doses than practitioner brands that are more targeted to specific issues.

4. Non-Medical Ingredients

Underneath the active ingredients list on most supplement labels there is a list of non-medical ingredients. These include fillers, binders, colours, flavours, and sweeteners. Be sure to check for these, as many of these ingredients can be irritating to your child.

You can also check my website for some brands I recommend.

Appendix J

Phenols in Food

In the discussion of food allergies in Part One, phenols were mentioned as a possible food trigger. Use the following lists to experiment with phenols reduction if any of those symptoms seemed relevant. Try eliminating the high and very high foods first, sticking with the low foods for about a week. If your child is sensitive to phenols you will see a reprieve in symptoms within a couple of days of reducing them. If phenols turn out to be a problem for your child, seek help with creating a nutritious low phenol diet and with addressing the underlying causes so phenols can be reintroduced. A low phenol diet can quickly becoming nutrient-poor as it is very restrictive. NOTE: The following list is not comprehensive, but it will give you a starting point.

Low Phenol Foods

Fruits: yellow apples, bananas, pears, pomegranates, mangos, papayas

Vegetables: asparagus, beets, bok choy, Brussels sprouts, butternut squash, cabbage, carrots, celery, green/string beans, lettuce, peas, potatoes, rutabagas, sweet potatoes, turnip

Nuts/Seeds: cashews, poppy seeds

Grains: arrowroot, buckwheat, millet, rice

Animal foods: beef, eggs, fish, lamb, liver, pork, poultry, shellfish

Other: carob powder, chives, cocoa powder, maple syrup, parsley, saffron, shallots, chamomile, garlic, salt, pure vanilla

High and Very High Phenol Foods

Fruits: apricots, blackberries, blueberries, boysenberries, cranberries, dates, guava, loganberries, avocados, raisins, prunes, strawberries, raspberries, apples, cantaloupe, cherries, grapes, raisins, currents, nectarines, peaches, oranges, pineapple

Vegetables: chicory, endive, peppers (red/yellow/green), mushrooms, radishes, tomatoes, zucchini, cucumbers, spinach, seaweed

Nuts: almonds, peanuts, water chestnuts

Grains: basmati rice, jasmine rice

Other: most spices including bay leaves, basil, caraway, chili powder, ginger root, mint, nutmeg, pepper, pimentos, allspice, cardamom, cloves, dill, licorice, paprika, aniseed, cayenne, celery powder, cinnamon, cumin, curry, dill, horseradish, mace, mustard, oregano, rosemary, sage, tarragon, turmeric, thyme; tea (green/black); vanilla flavouring (not pure); vinegar; Worchestershire sauce; honey; bacon, ham; bone broths; corn flour; fermented foods

Appendix K

Common Deficiency Symptoms

NOTE: This is not a diagnostic tool. No one symptom is enough to determine deficiency. Use your answers to start a conversation with your health care team about possible testing, supplementation, and diet strategy.

Deficiency	Symptom
B1	anxiety, irritability, fear apathy sleep disturbances poor coordination swelling weight loss or poor weight gain poor appetite
B2	dermatitis lack of taste cracked lips persistently watery or bloodshot eyes
B3	abdominal discomfort, nausea/diarrhea depression poor memory, confusion rough skin, skin lesions canker sores bad breath fatigue hypoglycemia
B5	fatigue burning or numb feet cramps abdominal discomfort acne poor coordination hair loss

Raising Resilience

B6		acne
		dermatitis
		muscle weakness
		irritability
		depression
		poor stress control
		poor immunity
		tooth decay
		fatigue
		anemia
		poor dream recall, stressful, bizarre dreams, nightmares
		strong reaction to alcohol and drugs
		light nausea in the morning
		motion sickness
		sensitivity to MSG
		sensitivity to light and sound
B12		poor memory
		prone to viral infections
		depression
		poor balance, clumsiness
		fatigue
		confusion
		poor sucking/swallowing
		delays in speech
		poor appetite
		failure to thrive
Biotin		muscle pain
		depression
		hair loss
		dermatitis
Copper		anemia
		depression
		fatigue
		hair loss
		bruising
		always feeling cold
		poor, stunted growth
Zinc		acne
		brittle nails
		depression, mood swings
		delayed puberty
		poor growth
		hair loss
		poor appetite, poor sense of taste/smell
		poor immunity

Appendices

	white spots on fingernails, paper thin nails
	joints popping, cracking, pain between shoulder blades, cartilage problems
	explosive temper, poor stress control
	poor short term memory
	depression
	frequent infections
	inability to tan
	poor dream recall
	crowded teeth, many cavities
	nervousness
	anxiety, inner tension
	bad breath and body odor (sweet, fruity)
	ringing in the ears
	sensitivity to metals
	poor concentration
Vitamin C	bleeding gums
	easy bruising, slow wound healing
	joint pain
	dry, splitting hair
	rough, dry skin
	nosebleeds
	chronic infections
Iron	anemia
	brittle nails
	confusion or poor memory
	headaches
	mouth/tongue sores
	fatigue, weakness
	pale skin
	cravings for non food items like ice or dirt
	irregular heart beat, shortness of breath
Chromium	anxiety
	fatigue
	slow growth
	sensitivity to carbohydrates
	hypoglycemia
	mood swings
Iodine	fatigue
	weight gain
	dry skin and hair, brittle nails
	puffy face
	poor memory
	depression
	constipation

Raising Resilience

Magnesium	muscle spasms insomnia hyperactivity restless legs teeth grinding headaches, migraines trouble detoxifying (chemical sensitivity) Raynaud's syndrome tooth decay hypoglycemia depression asthma constipation muscle spasms anxiety, panic attacks, poor stress control
Manganese	dizziness ringing in ears sensitivity to carbohydrates seizures mottled skin tone
Selenium	fatigue pancreatic insufficiency immune impairment
Sodium	cramps constipation PMS and morning sickness
Vitamin D	diarrhea insomnia seasonal depression sweating from the head poor coordination autoimmune conditions
Vitamin E	altered gait poor reflex dry, itchy skin
Calcium	brittle nails cramps depression tooth decay insomnia high soda intake
Vitamin K	bleeding ulcers nose bleeds

Appendices

	bruising liver or kidney disease
Vitamin A	night blindness acne dry skin and hair infertility poor growth sluggish immune system poor wound healing
Yeast	thrush chronic congestion bloating, gas sugar cravings eczema, psoriasis attention problems, difficulty concentrating, spacey anal itching unexplained fatigue weight gain, difficulty losing weight stimming, repetitive gestures, repeating phrases over and over toe-walking decreased eye contact inappropriate silly, goofy behaviour recurring cradle cap yellow and thick nails
Thyroid fatigue	low body temperature, cold all the time fatigue weight loss or weight gain slow growth recurrent infections depression anxiety poor concentration delayed development of permanent teeth hyperactivity fine motor problems forgetfulness low motivation anxious, depressed headaches constipation
Poor liver function	sensitive to perfumes, chemicals, cigarettes headaches, migraines poor appetite constipation eczema

	acne
	fatty stools
	abdominal pain after eating
Adrenal fatigue	persistent fatigue, especially sluggish on waking
	salt cravings
	lethargy
	decreased ability to handle stress
	frequent infections
	low stamina
	long recovery times
	depression, anxiety, fear
	hypoglycemia that doesn't respond to dietary changes
	environmental, chemical sensitivities
	poor memory, brain fog, difficulty concentrating
	allergies
	dizzy, especially when getting up from a lying down position

Appendix L

Glutamate and Additives

In the discussion of food allergies in Part One, glutamate was mentioned as a possible food trigger. Use the following lists to experiment with glutamate reduction if any of those symptoms seem relevant. If your child is sensitive to glutamate you will see a reprieve in symptoms within a couple of days of reducing them.

Glutamate-Rich Additives
- anything with glutamate in the name
- autolyzed yeast
- calcium caseinate or sodium caseinate
- carrageenan
- citric acid
- dextrose
- flavours or flavouring
- hydrolysed protein
- maltodextrin
- modified food starch
- monosodium glutamate (MSG)
- soy protein
- soy protein isolate
- textured vegetable protein
- whey protein (concentrate or isolate)
- xanthan gum
- yeast extract

Glutamate-Rich Foods

- barley malt
- broth or stock (even homemade)
- corn starch
- gelatin
- all dairy, especially parmesan cheese
- soy sauce
- fermented food
- bouillon
- brown rice syrup
- corn syrup
- milk powder
- rice syrup
- vegemite and marmite

Appendix M

Some Signs of Gut Dysbiosis

Digestive: bloating, excessive gas (particularly after eating carbohydrates like beans), pain, distention, persistent constipation, persistent diarrhea, indigestion, reflux, rectal itching, greasy stools, irritable bowel syndrome

Neurological: anxiety, depression, fatigue, insomnia, mood swings, hyperactivity, poor memory, spaciness, body aches, fatigue, low energy, reduced ability to handle stress

Immune: asthma, allergies, food sensitivities, chemical sensitivities, persistent infections, sluggish immune system, any diagnosed autoimmune disease

Skin/nails: eczema, psoriasis, persistent athlete's foot, nail fungus

Other: persistent iron or B12 deficiency, unexplained weight loss, any symptoms relating to malabsorption, chronic bad breath, strong body odor, persistent sinus congestion

Appendix N

Whole Foods to Have Handy

Milk and Substitutes	Butters	Meat/Fish
coconut milk (regular and light) 3.8% whole milk rice milk (Ryza if possible) unsweetened almond milk unsweetened kefir (or make your own) hemp milk	unsalted cultured butter sunflower seed butter tahini or sesame butter pumpkin seed butter almond butter macadamia nut butter	ground beef stewing cubes (beef, lamb) chicken (whole, with bones) liver (any kind) beef bones sardines (packed in water) wild Alaskan salmon with skin and bones (canned and fresh) whole fish with heads (for making broth) scallops, shrimp, oysters, clams
Beans	**Oils**	**Sweeteners**
chick-peas kidney beans black beans green/brown/red lentils split green peas blackeye peas great northern beans	coconut oil (refined or unrefined) flax oil olive oil unsalted butter sunflower oil ghee (or butter) red palm oil sesame oil	Sucanat or cane sugar unfiltered raw honey maple syrup blackstrap molasses coconut (palm) sugar rice syrup xylitol stevia coconut nectar
Grains	**Seeds/Nuts**	**Pasta**
millet quinoa long or short grain brown rice steel cut oats quick rolled oats amaranth buckwheat groats	flax seeds hemp seeds chia seeds sunflower seeds sesame seeds (white and black) pumpkin seeds walnuts almonds Brazil nuts	Kamut quinoa buckwheat rice whole wheat if gluten is okay (lasagne, macaroni, rotini, spaghetti)

Appendices

Fresh	Salt/Seasonings	Other
white potatoes and sweet potatoes eggs seasonal fruit (bananas, apples, kiwis, mangos, berries—not too much citrus) greens (chard, kale, spinach) butternut squash, pumpkin broccoli cauliflower carrots onions zucchini mushrooms (dried shitaki if you can find them) additional as per seasons	Himalayan salt unrefined sea salt garlic pure vanilla extract lemon juice umeboshi paste tamari (wheat-free, gold label) Worchestershire sauce (or make your own) fish sauce coconut aminos turmeric root ground: cumin, coriander, turmeric, cardamom, cinnamon, nutmeg, cloves, pepper, ginger, paprika, curry powder, pepper, fenugreek dried: dill, parsley, basil, thyme, sage, marjoram, oregano whole: bay leaf, peppercorns, cloves	apple sauce tortillas unfiltered apple cider vinegar wild salmon with skin and bones soft tofu (if tolerated) pita thin rice cakes frozen berries frozen mangos shredded coconut quinoa flakes mayonnaise (or make your own) nutritional yeast kelp powder Dijon mustard frozen green peas frozen corn diced tomato (or freeze in the fall!) dried kombu and wakame tomato paste crackers dulse flakes

Flours	Dried Fruit	Cheese
spelt, Kamut, rye, whole wheat (if gluten is tolerated) oat flour amaranth flour buckwheat flour chick-pea flour sorghum teff tapioca starch potato starch xanthan or guar gum (if gluten-free)	apricots figs dates raisins apples cranberries	mild cheddar shredded mozzarella soft goat's grated parmesan

REFERENCES

"Homeostasis." Dictionary.com. Unabridged. Random House, Inc. 2016. http://www.dictionary.com/browse/homeostasis.

"Resilience." Merriam-Webster.com. Last Accessed April 2016. http://www.merriam-webster.com/dictionary/resilience.

Morley, Wendy A. and Stephanie Seneff, *Diminished brain resilience syndrome: A modern day neurological pathology of increased susceptibility to mild brain trauma, concussion, and downstream neurodegeneration* "Surgical Neurology International (June 18, 2014), DOI: 10.4103/2152-7806. 134731.

ENDNOTES

1. "Aggression: a paradoxical response to tricyclic antidepressants," American Journal of Psychiatry 135 (January 28, 1978): 117–118. doi:10.1176/ajp.135.1.117; "Antidepressants linked to suicide and aggression in teens," U.S. National Library of Medicine (January 28, 2016), http://www.ncbi.nlm.nih.gov/pubmedhealth/behindtheheadlines/news/2016-01-28-antidepressants-linked-to-suicide-and-aggression-in-teens/.

2. Kate Johnson, "Antibiotic Exposure in Infancy Linked to Food Allergies," Medscape Medical News (February 28, 2013), http://www.medscape.com/viewarticle/780023; Mairi C. Noverr, Rachael M. Noggle, Galen B. Toews and Gary B. Huffnagle, "Role of Antibiotics and Fungal Microbiota in Driving Pulmonary Allergic Responses," American Society for Microbiology 72 (September 2004), http://iai.asm.org/content/72/9/4996.short.

3. AJ Henderson and SO Shaheen, "Acetaminophen and asthma," Paediatric Respiratory Reviews 14 (March 2013): 9–15, https://www.ncbi.nlm.nih.gov/pubmed/23347656.

4. Stephen T. Schultz et al, "Acetaminophen (paracetamol) use, measles-mumps-rubella vaccination, and autistic disorder," Sage Journals 12 (May 2008): 293–307, http://aut.sagepub.com/content/12/3/293.short.

5. Ragnhild Eek Brandlistuen et al, "Prenatal paracetamol exposure and child neurodevelopment: a sibling-controlled cohort study," International Journal of Epidemiology (October 24, 2013), doi:10.1093/ije/dyt183.

6. Zeyan Liew et al, "Acetaminophen Use During Pregnancy, Behavioral Problems, and Hyperkinetic Disorders," JAMA Pediatrics 168 (April 2014): 313–320, doi:10.1001/jamapediatrics.2013.4914.

7. AD Manthripragada et al, "Characterization of acetaminophen overdose-related emergency department visits and hospitalizations in the United States," Pharmacoepidemiology and Drug Safety 8 (August 20, 2011): 819–826, doi:10.1002/pds.2090.

8. Jeanne Van Cleave et al, "Dynamics of Obesity and Chronic Health Conditions Among Children and Youth," The JAMA Network 303 (February 17, 2010): 623–630, doi:10.10.1001/jama.2010.104; AS Gershon et al, "Trends in asthma prevalence and incidence in Ontario, Canada, 1996–2005: a population study," American Journal of Epidemiology 172 (September 15, 2010): 728–736, doi:10.1093/aje/kwq189; Eichenfield LF et al, "Atopic dermatitis and asthma: parallels in the evolution of treatment," Pediatrics 111 (2003): 608–616; SH Sicherer et al, "Prevalence of peanut and tree nut allergy in the United States determined by a random digit dial telephone survey: a 5-year follow-up study," The Journal of Allergy and Clinical Immunology 112 (2003): 1203–1207, doi:10.1016/S0091; Liam Delaney and James P. Smith,

"Children with Disabilities," *Princeton-Brookings* 22 (Spring 2012), http://www.futureofchildren.org/publications/journals/article/index.xml?journalid=77&articleid=560&sectionid=3874.

9. The term "microbiome" refers to the consortium of microbes that exist in our bodies. Throughout this book we will talk a lot about how these microbes influence our overall health.

10. J. Thirthalli et al, "Cortisol and antidepressant effects of yoga," *Indian Journal of Psychiatry* 55 (July 2013): S405–S408, doi:10.4103/0019-5545.116315; GH Naveen et al, "Positive therapeutic and neurotropic effects of yoga in depression: A comparative study," *Indian Journal of Psychiatry* 55 (2013): 400–404, http://indianjpsychiatry.org/article.asp?issn=0019-5545;year=2013;volume=55;issue=7;spage=400;epage=404;aulast=Naveen; BN Gangadhar et al, "Positive antidepressant effects of generic yoga in depressive outpatients: A comparative study," *Indian Journal of Psychiatry* 55 (August 2013): 369–373, http://indianjpsychiatry.org/article.asp?issn=0019-5545;year=2013;volume=55;issue=7;spage=369;epage=373;aulast=Gangadhar.

11. "Toxic Stress," *Center on the Developing Child, Harvard University*, http://developingchild.harvard.edu/science/key-concepts/toxic-stress/.

12. For more details on how the process of simplification affects resilience and behaviour look up the work of Kim John Payne - http://www.simplicityparenting.com/. For more details on the impact of school, family, peers and community on resilience see the work of Dr Wayne Hammond at the university of Calgary and the Resiliency Initative http://www.resil.ca/. Some great resources to better understand the impact of attachment on stress and behaviour look up the work of Gordon Neufeld http://neufeldinstitute.org/, and Todd Sarner -http://transformativeparenting.com/.

13. Martha Herbert and Cindy Sage, "Findings in Autism (ASD) Consistent with Electromagnetic Fields (EMF) and Radiofrequency Radiation (RFR)," *BioInitiative 2012* (2012), http://www.bioinitiative.org/report/wp-content/uploads/pdfs/sec20_2012_Findings_in_Autism.pdf.

14. Simon F. Thomsen, "Epidemiology and natural history of atopic diseases," *European Clinical Respiratory Journal* (March 24, 2015), doi:10.3402/ecri.v2.24642.

15. John Casey, "The Hidden Ingredient That Can Sabotage Your Diet," *MedicineNet.com*, http://www.medicinenet.com/script/main/art.asp?articlekey=56589.

16. "Added Sugars," *American Heart Association*, http://www.heart.org/HEARTORG/HealthyLiving/HealthyEating/Nutrition/Added-Sugars_UCM_305858_Article.jsp#.WD0CjrLx5hF.

17. Mary N. Haan, "Therapy Insight: type 2 diabetes mellitus and the risk of late-onset Alzheimer's disease," *Nature Reviews* (March 2006): 159–166, doi:10.1038/ncpneuro0124; Paula L. McClean et al, "Glucagon-like peptide-1 analogues enhance synaptic plasticity in the brain: A link between diabetes and Alzheimer's disease," *European Journal of Pharmacology* 630 (March 25, 2010): 158–162, doi.org/10.1016/j.ejphar.2009.12.023; Helaine E. Resnick and Barbara V. Howard, "Diabetes and Cardiovascular Disease," *Annual Reviews* 53 (February 2002): 245–267, doi:10.1146/annurev.med.53.082901.103904; Elizabeth Barrett-Connor, "Diabetes

Endnotes

and Heart Disease," *American Diabetes Association* 26 (October 2003): 2947–2958, doi.org/10.2337/diacare.26.10.2947; Scott M. Grundy et al, "Diabetes and Cardiovascular Disease," *AHA Scientific Statement* 100 (September 7, 1999): 1134–1146, doi.org/10.1161/01.CIR.100.10.1134; Paolo Vigneri et al, "Diabetes and cancer," *Society for Endocrinology* 16 (December 1, 2009): 1103–1123, doi:10.1677/ERC-09-0087; Zara Zelenko and Emily Jane Gallagher, "Diabetes and Cancer," *ScienceDirect* 43 (March 2014): 167–185, doi.org/10.1016/j.ecl.2013.09.008.

18. MS Diurhuus et al, "Insulin increases renal magnesium excretion: a possible cause of magnesium depletion in hyperinsulinaemic states," *Diabetic medicine: A Journal of the British Diabetic Association* 12 (August 1995): 664–669, https://www.ncbi.nlm.nih.gov/pubmed/7587003; J. Lemann Jr. et al, "Evidence that glucose ingestion inhibits net renal tubular reabsorption of calcium and magnesium in man," *Translational Research* 75 (April 1970): 578–585, http://www.translationalres.com/article/J2870%2990156-3/abstract; E. D'Erasmo et al, "Calcium homeostasis during oral glucose load in healthy women," *National Institute of Health* 31 (April 1999): 271–273, doi:10.1055/s-2007-978731; AS Kozlovsky et al, "Effects of diets high in simple sugars on urinary chromium losses," *National Institute of Health* 35 (June 1986): 515–518, https://www.ncbi.nlm.nih.gov/pubmed/3713513; John X. Wilson, "Regulation of vitamin C transport," *Annual Review of Nutrition* 25 (2005): 105–125, doi.org/10.1146/annurev.nutr.25.050304.092647.

19. G. Paolisso et al, "Daily magnesium supplements improve glucose handling in elderly subjects," *The American Journal of Clinical Nutrition* 55 (June 1992): 1161–1167, http://ajcn.nutrition.org/content/55/6/1161.abstract; Wilhelm Jahnen-Dechent and Markus Ketteler, "Magnesium basics," *Clinical Kidney Journal* 5 (2012): i3–i14, doi:10.1093/ndtplus/sfr163; R. Swaminathan, "Magnesium Metabolism and its Disorders," *The Clinical Biochemist Reviews* 24 (May 2003): 47–66, https://www.ncbi.nlm.nih.gov/pmc/articles/PMC1855626/; Carolyn Dean, *The Magnesium Miracle* (New York: Ballantine, 2007); L. Tosiello, "Hypomagnesemia and diabetes mellitus. A review of clinical implications," *Archives of Internal Medicine* 156 (June 10, 1996): 1143–1148, https://www.ncbi.nlm.nih.gov/pubmed/8639008?dopt=Abstract; John B. Vincent, "Elucidating a Biological Role for Chromium at a Molecular Level," *Accounts of Chemical Research* 33 (August 2000): 503–510, doi:10.1021/ar990073r.

20. Isabelle Aeberli et al, "Low to moderate sugar-sweetened beverage consumption impairs glucose and lipid metabolism and promotes inflammation in healthy young men: a randomized controlled trial," *The American Journal of Clinical Nutrition* 94 (August 2011): 479–485, doi: 10.3945/ajcn.111.013540; W. Kruis et al, "Effect of diets low and high in refined sugars on gut transit, bile acid metabolism, and bacterial fermentation," *British Society of Gastroenterology and BMJ* 32 (1991): 367–371, doi:10.1136/gut.32.4.367; Katherine Esposito et al, "Inflammatory Cytokine Concentrations Are Acutely Increased by Hyperglycemia in Humans," *American Heart Association* 106 (September 30, 2002): 2067–2072, http://circ.ahajournals.org/content/106/16/2067.short.

21. Stephanie Seneff, "Sulfate Deficiency in Neurological Disease Following Aluminum and Glyphosate Exposure," (June 2, 2015), hosted by Jessica Sherman, PDF of PowerPoint, (PDF Version); Anthony Samsel and Stephanie Seneff, "Glyphosate,

pathways to modern diseases II: Celiac sprue and gluten intolerance," *The Journal of Institute of Experimental Pharmacology of Slovak Academy of Sciences* 6 (March 2014): 159–184, doi.org/10.2478/intox-2013-0026; Anthony Samsel and Stephanie Seneff, "Glyphosate, pathways to modern diseases III: Manganese, neurological diseases, and associated pathologies," *Surgical Neurology International* 6 (March 24, 2015): 45, doi:10.4103/2152-7806.153876; Stephanie Seneff et al, "Aluminum and Glyphosate Can Synergistically Induce Pineal Gland Pathology: Connection to Gut Dysbiosis and Neurological Disease," *Agricultural Sciences* (January 2015): 42–70, http://search.proquest.com/openview/48f590b0e1f64663ea8a5470b9a452c7/1?pq-origsite=gscholar.

22. Anthony Samsel and Stephanie Seneff, "Glyphosate, pathways to modern diseases II: Celiac sprue and gluten intolerance," *The Journal of Institute of Experimental Pharmacology of Slovak Academy of Sciences* 6 (March 2014): 159–184, doi.org/10.2478/intox-2013-0026; Christopher A. Shaw et al, "Aluminum-Induced Entropy in Biological Systems: Implications for Neurological Disease," *Journal of Toxicology* (2014): Article 491316, doi.org/10.1155/2014/491316; Nancy L. Swanson et al, "Genetically engineered crops, glyphosate and the deterioration of health in the United States of America," *Journal of Organic Systems* 9 (2014), http://jeffreydachmd.com/wp-content/uploads/2015/04/Genetically-engineered-crops-glyphosate-deterioration-health-United-States-Swanson-J-Organic-Systems-2014.pdf; Stephanie Seneff et al, "Aluminum and Glyphosate Can Synergistically Induce Pineal Gland Pathology: Connection to Gut Dysbiosis and Neurological Disease," *Scientific Research* 6 (2015), doi:10.4236/as.2015.61005.

23. Kathryn Z. Guyton et al, " Carcinogenicity of Tetrachlorvinphos, Parathion Malathion, Diazinon, and Glyphosate." *The Lancet Oncology* 16 (May 2015): 490–491, doi.org/10.1016/S1470-2045(15)70134-8.

24. For a more complete download-able list of endocrine disruptors visit the Environmental Working Group http://www.ewg.org/research/dirty-dozen-list-endocrinedisruptors.

25. Tian Xia et al, "Quinones and Aromatic Chemical Compounds in Particulate Matter Induce Mitochondrial Dysfunction: Implications for Ultrafine Particle Toxicity," *Environmental Health Perspectives* 112 (October 14, 2004): 1347–1358, http://www.jstor.org/stable/3838072; Tian Xia et al, "Impairment of mitochondrial function by particulate matter (PM) and their toxic components: implications for PM-induced cardiovascular and lung disease," *Frontiers in Bioscience* 12 (February 2007): 1238–1246, doi:10.2741/2142.

26. Renato Polimanti et al, "Genetic variability of glutathione S-transferase enzymes in human populations: Functional inter-ethnic differences in detoxification systems," *ScienceDirect* 512 (January 2013): 102–107, doi.org/10.1016/j.gene.2012.09.113; Min Shi et al, "Orofacial Cleft Risk Is Increased with Maternal Smoking and Specific Detoxification-Gene Variants," *ScienceDirect* 80 (January 2007): 76–90, doi.org/10.1086/510518; Romilly E. Hodges and Deanna M. Minich, "Modulation of Metabolic Detoxification Pathways Using Foods and Food-Derived Components: A Scientific Review with Clinical Application," *Journal of Nutrition and Metabolism* (2015): Article 760689, doi:10.1155/2015/760689.

Endnotes

27. Ibid.

28. For more details about these concerns refer to the book and movie, Genetic Roulette here http://geneticroulettemovie.com/ the institute for Responsible Technology at http://responsibletechnology.org/ and GMwatch http://www.gmwatch.org/.

29. "The American Academy Of Environmental Medicine Calls For Immediate Moratorium On Genetically Modified Foods," *American Academy of Environmental Medicine* Media Release (May 19, 2009), https://www.aaemonline.org/gmo-pressrelease.php.

30. Corn, soy, sugar beets, canola, papaya, aspartame, cotton and some squashes are the crops that are currently routinely genetically modified. Apples, sweet corn, tomatoes, pigs and salmon are also slowly being introduced. Because many additives, synthetic hormones and most animal feed involve some combination of corn, soy and sugar, and because we have no labelling laws in place to indicate GM ingredients, most of us end up ingesting GM foods secondarily through additives, meat, dairy and eggs even if we are careful to avoid the crops that are modified directly.

31. J. Uittamo et al, "Xylitol inhibits carcinogenic acetaldehyde production by Candida species," *International Journal of Cancer* 129 (October 15, 2011): 2038–2041, doi:10.1002/ijc.25844.

32. Carolee Bateson-Koch, *Allergies Disease in Disguise* (Summertown: Books Alive, 1994), 77.

33. W. J. Delprado et al, "Placental candidiasis: report of three cases with a review of the literature," *National Institute of Health* 14 (April 1982): 191–195, https://www.ncbi.nlm.nih.gov/pubmed/7099725; Carolee Bateson-Koch, Allergies Disease in Disguise (Summertown: Books Alive, 1994).

34. The only way to know for sure if you are dealing with a yeast overgrowth is to have your doctor test either for it directly or for the metabolites it produces. You can find a great self assessment questionnaire at http://www.yeastconnection.com/yeast.html to get a sense of whether this might be a problem for your child.

35. Carolee Bateson-Koch, Allergies Disease in Disguise (Summertown: Books Alive, 1994).

36. Ben F. Feingold, "Hyperkinesis and Learning Disabilities Linked to Artificial Food Flavors and Colors," *American Journal of Nursing* 75 (May 1975), http://journals.lww.com/ajnonline/Abstract/1975/05000/Hyperkinesis_and_Learning_Disabilities_Linked_to.21.aspx.

37. Jeffrey A. Mattes, "The Feingold Diet, A Current Reappraisal," *Journal of Learning Disabilities* 16 (June/July 1983): 319–323, doi: 10.1177/002221948301600602.

38. Bernard Rimland, "The Feingold Diet: An Assessment of the Reviews by Mattes, by Kavale and Forness and Others," *Journal of Learning Disabilities* 16 (June/July 1983): 331–333, http://www.feingold.org/Research/rimland.html, www.feingold.org.

39. "Tylenol Fueling Autism Epidemic?" *Autism Coach*, http://autismcoach.com/tylenol-fueling-autism-epidemic/.

40. Bernard Rimland, "The Feingold Diet: An Assessment of the Reviews by Mattes, by Kavale and Forness and Others," *Journal of Learning Disabilities* 16 (June/July 1983): 331–333, http://orthomolecular.org/library/jom/1984/pdf/1984-v13n01-p045.pdf

41. S. Paruthi, "Recommended Amount of Sleep for Pediatric Populations: A Consensus Statement of the American Academy of Sleep Medicine," *Journal of Clinical Sleep Medicine* 12 (June 15, 2016): 785–786, doi:10.5664/jcsm.5866.

42. Rachel Leproult and Eve Van Cauter, "Role of Sleep and Sleep Loss in Hormonal Release and Metabolism," *US National Library of Medicine* (November 24, 2009), doi:10.1159/000262524.

43. Dieter Riemann, "Sleep and depression—results from psychobiological studies: an overview," *ScienceDirect* 57 (August 2001): 67–103, doi.org/10.1016/S0301-0511(01)00090-4.

44. Jane C. Evans et al, "Sleep and Healing in Intensive Care Settings," *Dimensions of Critical Care Nursing* 14 (July/August 1995), http://journals.lww.com/dccnjournal/abstract/1995/07000/sleep_and_healing_in_intensive_care_settings.5.aspx; R. Smith, "Recovery and Tissue Repair," *British Medical Bulletin* 41 (1985): 295–301, http://bmb.oxfordjournals.org/content/41/3/295.short.

45. Pierre Maquet, "The Role of Sleep in Learning and Memory," *Science* 294 (November 2001): 1048–1052, doi:10.1126/science.1062856; Giuseppe Curcio et al, "Sleep loss, learning capacity and academic performance," *Sleepmedicine Reviews* 10 (October 2006): 323–337, doi.org/10.1016/j.smrv.2005.11.001.

46. Neeraj K. Gupta et al, "Is obesity associated with poor sleep quality in adolescents?" *American Journal of Human Biology* 14 (November 2002): 762–768, doi:10.1002/ajhb.10093; Roland von Kanel et al, "Poor Sleep is Associated with Higher Plasma Proinflammatory Cytokine Interleukin-6 and Procoagulant Marker Fibrin D-Dimer in Older Caregivers of People with Alzheimer's Disease, " *Journal of the American Geriatrics Society* 54 (March 2006): 431–437, doi:10.1111/j.1532-5415.2005.00642.x; Anne B. Newman et al, "Sleep Disturbance, Psychosocial Correlates, and Cardiovascular Disease in 5201 Older Adults: The Cardiovascular Health Study," *Journal of the American Geriatrics Society* 45 (January 1997): 1–7, doi:10.1111/j.1532-5415.1997.tb00970.x.

47. K. Spiegel et al, "Brief communication: sleep curtailment in healthy young men is associated with decreased leptin levels, elevated ghrelin levels and increased hunger and appetite," *Annals of Internal Medicine* 141 (December 7, 2004): 846–850, https://www.ncbi.nlm.nih.gov/pubmed/15583226.

48. K. Spiegel et al, "Impact of sleep debt on metabolic and endocrine function," *Lancet* 354 (1999): 1435–1439, http://www.medscape.com/medline/abstract/10543671; A. N. Vgontzas et al, "Adverse effects of modest sleep restriction on sleepiness, performance, and inflammatory cytokines," *Medscape* 89 (2004): 2119–2126, http://www.medscape.com/medline/abstract/15126529; K. Spiegel et al, "Brief Communication: Sleep curtailment in healthy young men is associated with decreased leptin levels, elevated ghrelin levels and increased hunger and appetite," Annals of Internal Medicine 141 (December 7, 2004): 846–850, https://www.ncbi.nlm.nih.gov/pubmed/15583226.

Endnotes

49. James B. Adams and Charles Holloway, "Pilot Study of a Moderate Dose Multivitamin/Mineral Supplement for Children with Autistic Spectrum Disorder," *The Journal of Alternative and Complementary Medicine* 10 (2004): 1033–1039, http://www.brainchildnutritionals.com/lanotattachments/download/file/id/3/store/1/arizonastudy.pdf; James B. Adams et al, "Effect of a vitamin/mineral supplement on children and adults with autism," *BMC Pediatrics* 11 (2011): 111, doi.org/10.1186/1471-2431-11-111; Julie Matthews, *Nourishing Hope for Autism: Nutrition Intervention for Healing Our Children* (Healthful Living Media, 2008); James B. Adams, "Vitamin/Mineral Supplements for Children and Adults with Autism," *Vitamins & Minerals* 4 (2015), doi:10.4172/2376-1318.1000127.

50. Michael R. Lyon, *Is Your Child's Brain Starving?* (2002); L. J. Stevens et al, "Essential fatty acid metabolism in boys with attention-deficit hyperactivity disorder," *The American Journal of Clinical Nutrition* 62 (October 1995): 761–768, http://ajcn.nutrition.org/content/62/4/761.short; Alexandra J. Richardson and Basant K. Pun, "A randomized double-blind, placebo-controlled study of the effects of supplementation with highly unsaturated fatty acids on ADHD-related symptoms in children with specific learning difficulties," *ScienceDirect* 26 (February 2002): 233–239, doi.org/10.1016/S0278-5846(01)00254-8; M. H. Bloch and A. Qawasmi, "Omega-3 fatty acid supplementation for the treatment of children with attention-deficit/hyperactivity disorder symptomatology: systematic review and meta-analysis," *Journal of the American Academy of Child and Adolescent Psychiatry* 50 (October 2011): 991–1000, doi:10.1016/j.jaac.2011.06.008; A. J. Richardson and B. K. Puri, "A randomized double-blind, placebo-controlled study of the effects of supplementation with highly unsaturated fatty acids on ADHD-related symptoms in children with specific learning difficulties," *US National Library of Medicine* 26 (February 2002): 233–239, https://www.ncbi.nlm.nih.gov/pubmed/11817499; N. Sinn and J. Bryan, "Effect of supplementation with polyunsaturated fatty acids and micronutrients on learning and behavior problems associated with child ADHD," *US National Library of Medicine* 28 (April 2007): 82–91, https://www.ncbi.nlm.nih.gov/pubmed/17435458.

51. V. Lobo et al, "Free radicals, antioxidants and functional foods: Impact on human health," *Pharmacognosy Review* 4 (July-December 2010): 118–126, doi:10.4103/0973-7847.70902.

52. Asli Sarandol et al, "Major depressive disorder is accompanied with oxidative stress: short-term antidepressant treatment does not alter oxidative-antioxidative systems," *Wiley Online Library* (February 14, 2007), doi:10.1002/hup.829.

53. Nidhin Joseph et al, "Oxidative Stress and ADHD: A Meta-Analysis," *Journal of Attention Disorders* (November 14, 2013), doi:10.1177/1087054713510354.

54. "Pollution in Minority Newborns," *EWG.org* (November 23, 2009), http://www.ewg.org/research/minority-cord-blood-report/executive-summary.

55. Environmental Defence, "PRE-POLLUTED: A report on the toxic substances in the umbilical cord blood of Canadian newborns," *Environmental Defence* (June 2013), http://environmentaldefence.ca/report/report-pre-polluted-a-report-on-toxic-substances-in-the-umbilical-cord-blood-of-canadian-newborns/.

56. Emily J. McAllister et al, "Ten Putative Contributors to the Obesity Epidemic," *Critical Reviews in Food Science and Nutrition* 49 (2009): doi.org/10.1080/10408390903372599; Peter J. Turnbaugh et al, "A core gut microbiome in obese and lean twins," *Nature* 457 (January 22, 2009): 480–484, doi:10.1038/nature07540; Peter J. Turnbaugh et al, "An obesity-associated gut microbiome with increased capacity for energy harvest," *Nature* 444 (December 21, 2006): 1027–1031, doi:10.1038/nature05414; Peter J. Turnbaugh et al, "Diet-Induced Obesity is Linked to Marked but Reversible Alterations in the Mouse Distal Gut Microbiome," *ScienceDirect* 3 (April 17, 2008): 213–223, doi.org/10.1016/j.chom.2008.02.015; J. L. Tang-Péronard et al, "Endocrine-disrupting chemicals and obesity development in humans: A review," *Wiley Online Library* (April 4, 2011), doi:10.1111/j.1467-789X.2011.00871.x; Roya Kelishadi et al, "Role of Environmental Chemicals in Obesity: A Systematic Review on the Current Evidence," *Journal of Environmental and Public Health* 2013 (2013), Article 896789, doi.org/10.1155/2013/896789; David S. Ludwig et al, "Relation between consumption of sugar-sweetened drinks and childhood obesity: a prospective, observational analysis," *The Lancet* 357 (February 17, 2001): 505–508, doi.org/10.1016/S0140-6736(00)04041-1.

57. "Intake Recommendations," *Nutri-Facts*, http://www.nutri-facts.org/content/nutrifacts/en_US/nutrients/essential-fatty-acids/essential-fatty-acids/intake-recommendations.html; Joseph R. Hibbeln et al, "Healthy intakes of n-3 and n-6 fatty acids: estimations considering worldwide diversity," *The American Journal of Clinical Nutrition* 83 (June 2006): S 1483–1493S, http://ajcn.nutrition.org/content/83/6/S1483.abstract; PM Kris-Etherton et al, "Polyunsaturated fatty acids in the food chain in the United States," *The American Journal of Clinical Nutrition* 7 (January 2000): 179S–188S, http://ajcn.nutrition.org/content/71/1/179S.full?ijkey=5c7af875f3dc71a303f7df78c52145e8b7c31643; G. L. Russo, "Dietary n-6 and n-3 polyunsaturated fatty acids: from biochemistry to clinical implications in cardiovascular prevention," *US National Library of Medicine* 77 (March 15, 2009): 937–946, doi:10.1016/j.bcp.2008.10.020.

58. "Effect of Zinc Deficiency on Blood Glutathione Levels," *The Journal of Nutrition* 111 (June 1, 1981): 1098–1102, http://jn.nutrition.org/content/111/6/1098.full.pdf.

59. J. DiFrancisco-Donoghue et al, "Effects of exercise and B vitamins on homocysteine and glutathione in Parkinson's disease: a randomized trial," *US National Library of Medicine* 10 (2012): 127–134, dio:10.1159/000333790.

60. E. Garcion et al, "New clues about vitamin D functions in the nervous system," *US National Library of Medicine* 13 (April 2002): 100–105, https://www.ncbi.nlm.nih.gov/pubmed/11893522.

61. Monica H. Carlsen et al, "The total antioxidant content of more than 3100 foods, beverages, spices, herbs and supplements used worldwide," *Nutrition Journal* 9 (January 22, 2010), doi:10.1186/1475-2891-9-3.

62. Ron Sender et al, "Revised estimates for the number of human and bacteria cells in the body," *bioRxiv* (January 6, 2016), dx.doi.org/10.1101/036103.

Endnotes

63. Augusto J. Montiel-Castro et al, "The microbiota-gut-brain axis: neurobehavioral correlates, health and sociality," *Frontiers in Integrative Neuroscience* 7 (October 7, 2013), doi:10.3389/fnint.2013.00070.

64. Ibid.

65. O. O. Oquntibeju et al, "Red palm oil: nutritional, physiological and therapeutic roles in improving human wellbeing and quality of life," *British Journal of Biomedical Science* 66 (2009): 216–222, https://www.ncbi.nlm.nih.gov/pubmed/20095133.

66. Philippe Grandjean and Philip J. Landrigan, "Neurobehavioural effects of developmental toxicity," *The Lancet* 13 (March 2014): 330–338, doi.org/10.1016/S1474-4422(13)70278-3; Megan Brooks, "Organophosphate Pesticides Linked to ADHD," *Medscape* (May 17, 2010), http://www.medscape.com/viewarticle/721892; Maryse F. Bouchard et al, "Attention-Deficit/Hyperactivity Disorder and Urinary Metabolites of Organophosphate Pesticides," *Pediatrics* 125 (June 2010), http://pediatrics.aappublications.org/content/125/6/e1270.abstract; Lu Chensheng et al, "Organic Diets Significantly Lower Children's Dietary Exposure to Organophosphorus Pesticides," *Environmental Health Perspectives* 114 (February 2006): 260–263, doi:10.1289/ehp.8418.

67. Sometimes blood sugar testing is misleading. Reactive hypoglycemia is a condition in which symptoms of low blood sugar are present but blood sugar levels read within a normal range. These kids will have a strong sugar reaction when they ingest simple carbohydrates because an overproduction of insulin plummets their blood sugar and causes the release of epinephrine, but it is harder to detect via testing.

68. Timothy W. Jones et al, "Independent Effects of Youth and Poor Diabetes Control on Responses to Hypoglycemia in Children," *American Diabetes Association* 40 (March 1991): 358–363, doi.org/10.2337/diab.40.3.358.

69. H. C. Lukaski, "Chromium as a supplement," *Annual Review of Nutrition* 19 (1999): 279–302, doi:10.1146/annurev.nutr.19.1.279.

70. K. L. Johnston et al, "Resistant starch improves insulin sensitivity in metabolic syndrome," *Wiley Online Library* (April 7, 2010), doi:10.1111/j.1464-5491.2010.02923.x; Kevin C. Maki et al, "Resistant Starch from High-Amylose Maize Increases Insulin Sensitivity in Overweight and Obese Men," *The Journal of Nutrition* (February 22, 2012), doi:10.3945/jn.111.152975.

71. Danielle Alexander, "Postprandial effects of resistant starch corn porridges on blood glucose and satiety responses in non-overweight and overweight adults," *Iowa State University Digital Repository* (2012), Graduate Theses and Dissertations, http://lib.dr.iastate.edu/cgi/viewcontent.cgi?article=3729&context=etd; A. Raben et al, "Resistant starch: the effect on postprandial glycemia, hormonal response, and satiety," *The American Journal of Clinical Nutrition* 60 (October 1994): 544–551, http://ajcn.nutrition.org/content/60/4/544.short.

72. Furio Brighenti et al, "Colonic fermentation of indigestible carbohydrates contributes to the second-meal effect," *The American Journal of Clinical Nutrition* 83 (April 2006): 817–822, http://ajcn.nutrition.org/content/83/4/817.abstract.

73. Robert H. Lustig et al, "Public health: The toxic truth about sugar," *Nature* 482 (February 2, 2012): 27–29, doi:10.1038/482027a.

74. James S. Ruff et al, "Compared to Sucrose, Previous Consumption of Fructose and Glucose Monosaccharides Reduces Survival and Fitness of Female Mice," *The Journal of Nutrition* (2014), doi:10.3945/jn.114.202531.

75. "Sugar: The Bitter Truth," *University of California Television (UCTV)*, YouTube https://www.youtube.com/watch?v=dBnniua6-oM&feature=youtu.be.

76. "Caution on Fructose Consumption: Do This and You'll Likely Gain 15 Pounds Next Year," *Mercola.com* (January 3, 2011), http://articles.mercola.com/sites/articles/archive/2011/01/03/high-fructose-corn-syrup-even-worse-than-weve-been-told.aspx.

77. P. A. S. Theophilus et al, "Effectiveness of Stevia Rebaudiana Whole Leaf Extract Against the Various Morphological Forms of Borrelia Burgdorferi in Vitro," *European Journal of Microbiology & Immunology* 5 (December 2015): 268–280, doi:10.1556/1886.2015.00031.

78. J. Uittamo et al, "Xylitol inhibits carcinogenic acetaldehyde production by Candida species," *International Journal of Cancer* 129 (October 15, 2011): 2038–2041, doi:10.1002/ijc.25844.

79. K. O. Bushara, "Neurologic presentation of celiac disease," *US National Library of Medicine* 128 (April 2005): S92–S97, https://www.ncbi.nlm.nih.gov/pubmed/15825133; Hugh J. Freeman, "Neurological disorders in adult celiac disease," *Canadian Journal of Gastroenterology* 22 (November 2008): 909–911, https://www.ncbi.nlm.nih.gov/pmc/articles/PMC2661192/; Aaron Lerner et al, "Neurological Manifestations of Celiac Disease in Children and Adults," *European Neurological Journal* (2010), http://drperlmutter.com/wp-content/uploads/2013/07/CELIAC-CHILDREN-NEUROLOGICAL.pdf.

80. F. L. Soares et al, "Gluten-free diet reduces adiposity, inflammation and insulin resistance associated with the induction of PPAR-alpha and PPAR-gamma expression," *The Journal of Nutritional Biochemistry* 24 (June 2013): 1105–1111, doi:10.1016/j.jnutbio.2012.08.009; N. G. Cascella et al, "Prevalence of celiac disease and gluten sensitivity in the United States clinical antipsychotic trials of intervention effectiveness study population," *Schizophrenia Bulletin* 37 (January 2011): 94–100, doi:10.1093/schbul/sbp055; Nga M. Lau et al, "Markers of Celiac Disease and Gluten Sensitivity in Children with Autism," *PLOS One* (June 18, 2013), doi.org/10.1371/journal.pone.0066155; Jonas F. Ludvigsson et al, "Small-Intestinal Histopathology and Mortality Risk in Celiac Disease," *The JAMA Network* 302 (September 16, 2009): 1171–1178, doi:10.1001/jama.2009.1320; Alberto Rubio-Tapia et al, "Increased Prevalence and Mortality in Undiagnosed Celiac Disease," *ScienceDirect* 137 (July 2009): 88–93, doi.org/10.1053/j.gastro.2009.03.059; P. Margutti et al, "Autoantibodies associated with psychiatric disorders," *US National Library of Medicine* 3 (May 2006): 149–157, https://www.ncbi.nlm.nih.gov/pubmed/16719797; Khalafalla O. Bushara, "Neurologic presentation of celiac disease," *Gastroenterology* 128 (April 2005): S92–S97, doi.org/10.1053/j.gastro.2005.02.018; Richard J. Farrell and

Endnotes

Ciaran P. Kelly, "Celiac Sprue," *The New England Journal of Medicine* 346 (January 17, 2002): 180–188, doi:10.1056/NEJMra010852.

81. Karin de Punder and Leo Pruimboom, "The Dietary Intake of Wheat and other Cereal Grains and Their Role in Inflammation," *MDPI* 5 (March 2013): 771–787, doi:10.3390/nu5030771.

82. Sally Fallon, *Nourishing Traditions: The Cookbook that Challenges Politically Correct Nutrition and the Diet Dictocrats*, (Washington DC: NewTrends Publishing, 2001).

83. "Arsenic – what you need to know," *Greener Choices Consumer Reports*, http://greenerchoices.org/2016/02/04/arsenic/.

84. Ke-Yong Wang et al, "Histamine Regulation in Glucose and Lipid Metabolism via Histamine Receptors," *The American Journal of Pathology* 177 (August 2010): 713–723, doi:10.2353/ajpath.2010.091198.

85. "So What's the Big Deal about Food Allergies?" *Kids with Food Allergies*, http://www.kidswithfoodallergies.org/page/whats-the-big-deal-about-food-allergies.aspx.

86. "Food Allergy," *National Institute of Allergy and Infectious Diseases*, https://www.niaid.nih.gov/diseases-conditions/food-allergy.

87. "Allergy Statistics," *American Academy of Allergy Asthma & Immunology*, http://www.aaaai.org/about-aaaai/newsroom/allergy-statistics.

88. "The Global Asthma Report," *The Global Asthma Network* (2014), http://www.globalasthmareport.org/resources/Global_Asthma_Report_2014.pdf.

89. "Connection Between Allergic Diseases and Autoimmune Diseases," *ScienceDaily* (April 6, 2007), https://www.sciencedaily.com/releases/2007/04/070403161855.htm.

90. Andrew T. Stefka et al, "Commensal bacteria protect against food allergen sensitization," *National Academy of Sciences of the United States of America* 111 (June 25, 2014): 13145–13150, doi:10.1073/pnas.1412008111; Scarlet M. Salas et al, "Infant gut microbiota and the development of wheeze in early childhood," *Allergy, Asthma & Clinical Immunology* 10 (2014), doi:10.1186/1710-1492-10-S1-A35.

91. Malin R. Karlsson et al, "Allergen-responsive CD4+CD25+ Regulatory T Cells in Children who Have Outgrown Cow's Milk Allergy," *JEM* 199 (June 21, 2004): 1679–1688, doi:10.1084/jem.20032121.

92. S. L. Prescott and B. Björkstén, "Probiotics for the prevention or treatment of allergic diseases," *The Journal of Allergy and Clinical Immunology* 120 (August 2007): 255–262, https://www.ncbi.nlm.nih.gov/pubmed/17544096; J. Wassenberg et al, "Effect of Lactobacillus paracasei ST11 on a nasal provocation test with grass pollen in allergic rhinitis," *Journal of the British Society for Allergy and Clinical Immunology* 41 (April 2011): 565–573, doi:10.1111/j.1365-2222.2011.03695.x; D. J. Costa et al, "Efficacy and safety of the probiotic Lactobacillus paracasei LP-33 in allergic rhinitis: a double-blind, randomized, placebo-controlled trial (GA2LEN Study)," *European Journal of Clinical Nutrition* 68 (May 2014): 602–607, doi:10.1038/ejcn.2014.13; T. Y. Lin et al, "Effect of probiotics on allergic rhinitis in Df, Dp or dust-sensitive children: a randomized double blind controlled trial," *Indian Pediatrics* 50 (February 2013): 209–213, https://www.ncbi.nlm.nih.gov/pubmed/22728633.

93. Minna-Maija Grölund et al, "Fecal Microflora in Healthy Infants Born by Different Methods of Delivery: Permanent Changes in Intestinal Flora After Cesarean Delivery," *Journal of Pediatric Gastroenterology and Nutrition* 28 (January 1999): 19–25, http://journals.lww.com/jpgn/Abstract/1999/01000/Fecal_Microflora_in_Healthy_Infants_Born_by.7.aspx; Giacomo Biasucci et al, "Cesarean Delivery May Affect the Early Biodiversity of Intestinal Bacteria," *The Journal of Nutrition* 138 (September 2008): 1796S–1800S, http://jn.nutrition.org/content/138/9/1796S.short; John Penders et al, "Factors Influencing the Composition of the Intestinal Microbiota in Early Infancy," *Pediatrics* 118 (August 2006), http://pediatrics.aappublications.org/content/118/2/511.short; Hedvig E. Jakobsson et al, "Decreased gut microbiota diversity, delayed Bacteroidetes colonisation and reduced Th1 responses in infants delivered by Caesarean section," *Gut* 63 (2014): 559–566, doi:10.1136/gutjnl-2012-303249.

94. Evalotte Decker et al, "Cesarean Delivery Is Associated With Celiac Disease but Not Inflammatory Bowel Disease in Children," *Pediatrics* 125 (June 2010), http://pediatrics.aappublications.org/content/125/6/e1433.short; Mette C. Tollanes et al, "Cesarean Section and Risk of Severe Childhood Asthma: A Population-Based Cohort Study," *ScienceDirect* 153 (July 2008): 112–116, http://www.sciencedirect.com/science/article/pii/S002234760800070X; Peter Bager et al, "Mode of delivery and risk of allergic rhinitis and asthma," *ScienceDirect* 111 (January 2003): 51–56, http://www.sciencedirect.com/science/article/pii/S0091674902912960.

95. H. Chasiotis and S. P. Kelly, "Effect of cortisol on permeability and tight junction protein transcript abundance in primary cultured gill epithelia from stenohaline goldfish and euryhaline trout," *US National Library of Medicine* 172 (July 2011): 494–504, doi:10.1016/j.ygcen.2011.04.023; A. M. Sandbichler et al, "Cortisol affects tight junction morphology between pavement cells of rainbow trout gills in single-seeded insert culture," *US National Library of Medicine* 181 (December 2011): 1023–1034, doi:10.1007/s00360-011-0586-y.

96. Simon R. Knowles et al, "Investigating the role of perceived stress on bacterial flora activity and salivary cortisol secretion: A possible mechanism underlying susceptibility to illness," *ScienceDirect* 77 (February 2008): 132–137, http://www.sciencedirect.com/science/article/pii/S0301051107001597.

97. S. Noda et al, "Differential effects of flavonoids on barrier integrity in human intestinal Caco-2 cells," *Journal of Agricultural and Food Chemistry* 60 (May 9, 2012): 4628–4633, doi:10.1021/jf300382h; R. V. Espley et al, "Dietary flavonoids from modified apple reduce inflammation markers and modulate gut microbiota in mice," *The Journal of Nutrition* 144 (February 2014): 146–154, doi: 10.3945/jn.113.182659; Kanti Bhooshan Pandey and Syed Ibrahim Rizvi, "Plant polyphenols as dietary antioxidants in human health and disease," *Oxidative Medicine and Cellular Longevity* 2 (November-December 2009): 270–278, doi:10.4161/oxim.2.5.9498.

98. Ibid.

99. T. Morita et al, "Dietary resistant starch alters the characteristics of colonic mucosa and exerts a protective effect on trinitrobenzene sulfonic acid-induced colitis in rats,"

Endnotes

US National Library of Medicine 68 (October 2004): 2155–2164, doi:10.1271/bbb.68.2155.

100. Ellyn Satter, "Eating Competence: Definition and Evidence for the Satter Eating Competence Model," *Journal of Nutrition* 39 (2007): S142–S153, http://ellynsatterinstitute.org/cms-assets/documents/101150-596171.ecdefandev.pdf; For some criteria that determines a competent eater visit http://ellynsatterinstitute.org/cms-assets/documents/171739-623167.ecsi2withscoringandinterpretation.pdf.

101. Barbara Lohse et al, "Eating competence of elderly Spanish adults is associated with a healthy diet and a favorable cardiovascular disease risk profile," *The Journal of Nutrition* 140 (July 2010): 1322–1327, http://jn.nutrition.org/content/140/7/1322.short; Barbara Lohse et al, "Evaluation of About Being Active, an online lesson about physical activity shows that perception of being physically active is higher in eating competent low-income women," *BMC Women's Health* 13 (2013), doi:10.1186/1472-6874-13-12.

102. Virginia Quick et al, "Eat, Sleep, Work, Play: Associations of Weight Status and Health-Related Behaviors among Young Adult College Students," *American Journal of Health Promotion* 29 (November 2014), doi:10.4278/ajhp.130327-QUAN-130; Jodi Stotts Krall and Barbara Lohse, "Cognitive Testing with Female Nutrition and Education Assistance Program Participants Informs Validity of the Satter Eating Competence Inventory," *ScienceDirect* 42 (July-August 2010): 277–283, doi.org/10.1016/j.jneb.2009.08.003.

103. Barbara Lohse et al, "Evaluation of About Being Active, an online lesson about physical activity shows that perception of being physically active is higher in eating competent low-income women," *BMC Women's Health* 13 (2013), doi:10.1186/1472-6874-13-12.

104. Virginia Quick et al, "Eat, Sleep, Work, Play: Associations of Weight Status and Health-Related Behaviors among Young Adult College Students," *American Journal of Health Promotion* 29 (November 2014), doi:10.4278/ajhp.130327-QUAN-130.

105. Lohse, "Diet quality is related to eating competence in cross-sectional sample of low income females surveyed in Pennsylvania," *Appetite* 58 (April 2012): 645–650, https://www.ncbi.nlm.nih.gov/pubmed/22142509; Lohse, "Eating competence of elderly Spanish adults is associated with a healthy diet and a favorable cardiovascular disease risk profile," *The Journal of Nutrition* 140 (July 2010): 1322–1327, https://www.ncbi.nlm.nih.gov/pubmed/20505016; Lohse, "Measuring eating competence: psychometric properties and validity of the ecSatter Inventory," *The Journal of Nutrition* 39 (Sept-Oct. 2007): S154–166, https://www.ncbi.nlm.nih.gov/pubmed/17826696.

106. Tylka, "Which adaptive maternal eating behaviors predict child feeding practices? An examination with mothers of 2- to 5-year-old children," *Eat Behav* 14 (January 2013): 57–63, https://www.ncbi.nlm.nih.gov/pmc/articles/PMC3719163/; Barbara Lohse et al, "Development of a Tool To Assess Adherence to a Model of the Division of Responsibility in Feeding Young Children: Using Response Mapping To Capacitate

107. Eisenberg, "Correlations Between Family Meals and Psychosocial Well-being Among Adolescents," *Arch Pediatr Adolesc Med* 158 (August 2004): 792–796, doi:10.1001/archpedi.158.8.792.

108. Bananalink.org, "All about bananas," *Banana Link* (2016), http://www.bananalink.org.uk/all-about-bananas.

109. Stolarczyk, "Carrot: History and Iconography," *Chronica Horticulturae* 51 (2011): 13–18, http://www.carrotmuseum.co.uk/today.html.

110. CIP International Potato Center, "Potato Facts and Figures," *CIP Newsletter*, http://cipotato.org/potato/facts/.

111. Satter, "The Quest for Children's Food Acceptance," *Journal of the Academy of Nutrition and Dietetics* 113 (April 2013): 508–509, http://www.ellynsatterinstitute.org/cms-assets/documents/106962-811788.blissettletter.pdf.

112. Whiteley, "Biochemical aspects in autism spectrum disorders: updating the opioidexcess theory and presenting new opportunities for biomedical intervention," *Expert Opinion on Therapeutic Targets* 6 (2002), http://www.tandfonline.com/doi/abs/10.1517/14728222.6.2.175.

113. Satter, "Eating Competence: definition and evidence for the Satter Eating Competence Model," *J Nutr Edu Behav* 39 (2007): S142–S153, www.ellynsatterinstitute.org/cms-assets/documents/101150-596171.ecdefandev.pdf.

114. Walter, "Impact of iron deficiency on cognition in infancy and childhood," *European Journal of Clinical Nutrition* 47 (1993): 307–316; Grantham-McGregor, "A Review of Studies on the Effect of Iron Deficiency on Cognitive Development in Children," *The Journal of Nutrition* 131 (February 1, 2001), http://jn.nutrition.org/content/131/2/649S.full.

115. Konofal, "Effects of iron supplementation on attention deficit hyperactivity disorder in children," *US National Library of Medicine* 38 (January 2008), https://www.ncbi.nlm.nih.gov/pubmed/18054688; Konofal, "Iron Deficiency in Children With Attention-Deficit/Hyperactivity Disorder," *Arch Pediatr Adolesc Med* 158 (2004): 1113–1115, http://www.taylorbugkisses.com/Iron%20Deficiency%20with%20ADHD.pdf; Waknine, "Iron Supplementation May Help Children With ADHD," *Medscape* (December 6, 2004), http://www.medscape.com/viewarticle/495332.

116. Fallon, "Vitamin A Sage," *The Weston A. Price Foundation* (March 30, 2001), http://www.westonaprice.org/health-topics/abcs-of-nutrition/vitamin-a-saga/.

MORE ABOUT THE AUTHOR

Jess Sherman first became interested in the topic of physical and mental resilience as a high school teacher. Her concern about the growing number of students struggling with recurrent illness and infection, aberrant behaviour, blunted energy, sleep disorders, learning, and mental health challenges, compelled her back to school to study holistic health and nutrition.

Since 2007, in order to support her clients and the health and resilience of her own family, Jess has pursued additional training in digestive health, autism spectrum disorders, traditional food preparation, yoga and stress management, biological approaches to mental health, functional medicine, and has become board certified in practical holistic nutrition. Her training, along with her front-line work supporting families with autism, ADHD, and mental illness are what brought Jess to the compelling insights she delivers in Raising Resilience.

Permissions

Every attempt has been made to give proper acknowledgment, and access appropriate permissions for quotes. Any oversights are purely unintentional. In the unlikely event something has been missed, please accept our regret and apology, and contact us immediately so we can investigate and rectify as needed.

Publisher's Note

Raising Resilience is chock full of helpful, cutting-edge insights and recommendations you can use immediately. When you want to delve a little deeper Jess Sherman provides that as well, to help us fully comprehend the critical impact and importance of our family's nutrition and our approach to it.

As we comprehend the basics of any topic more questions often arise, taking us on a journey of wanting to learn more, especially when it comes to caring for our children. Author, Jess Sherman has gone above and beyond in *Raising Resilience*, generously sharing the benefits of her tireless study, committed research, and passion for living life with great health and vitality, and helping us do the same.

She uniquely understands how busy and sometimes challenging it can be raising a young family and has taken this into consideration in every single bit of knowledge, advice, and recipes she imparts.

Whether you need quick go-to notes and tips for feeding your family or a high level resource book, you will find it in *Raising Resilience*—and you will absolutely love having it all in one place.

It's been a joy to work with Jess and partner with her to bring *Raising Resilience* to life. We greatly admire her exceptional conscientiousness, and know that the ripple effect of this work will be solid and long-lasting.

Sheri Andrunyk
Publisher, Author, Speaker, Mentor
Insightful Communications (I C) Publishing
Committed to Quality Content, Design, and Platform

ICPublishing.ca / ICBookstore.ca

Made in United States
North Haven, CT
13 February 2022